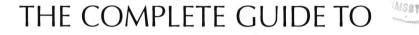

THE COMPLETE GUIDE TO

Strength Training

Anita Bean

0713643897

A & C Black • Lond

First published 1997 by
A & C Black (Publishers) Ltd
35 Bedford Row, London WC1R 4JH

Reprinted 1998, 1999

ISBN 0 7136 4389 7

A CIP catalogue record for this book
is available from the British Library.

Acknowledgments
The author would like to thank Simon Bean, Jon Cossins and
Peggy Wellington for their help with checking the manuscript.
Cover photograph courtesy of Jump, Hamburg.
All other photographs by Damian Walker. Location: Pavillion
Sports and Fitness Club, East Molesey, Surrey; clothing and
footwear supplied by Reebok and Puma.
Line diagrams on pages 17 and 29 by Jean Ashley.

Printed and bound in Great Britain by
WBC Book Manufacturers Ltd.

Contents

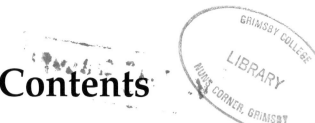

Introduction

Nutrition and strength training are equally important for making significant gains in strength, muscle mass and muscle definition. One without the other will result in slow progress or none at all. This book draws together the latest information on sports nutrition and scientifically-proven training methods, and tailors it to your particular goals. It will ensure that you optimise your progress.

Your basic body shape is determined by your genetic make-up and hormonal balance. However, everyone can improve their natural body shape through the right type of training programme and nutrition plan. Here you will find descriptions of the most common body types and shapes, and outlines of strategies for improving your shape.

You will also find explanations of the scientific principles behind strength training: how muscles become stronger and increase in size and mass; why some people respond more readily to strength training than others; how the proportion of different muscle fibre types influences your ability to develop strength or endurance; how you can make the fastest possible progress towards your goals.

There are training programmes for both beginners and advanced trainers. You can make continual improvements and avoid reaching plateaux by applying new methods such as eccentric training to stimulate maximum muscle growth and also by using training cycles throughout the year. The book also reveals the latest evidence on optimal rest periods, recovery and advanced training techniques.

Muscle definition is a major goal for many trainers and sports-people and this is achieved by increasing muscle mass and reducing body fat. Research indicates that everyone has a genetically determined percentage fat range which the body strives to maintain even when dieting or overeating. My manual presents dietary and training strategies for losing body fat, gaining lean mass and preparing for competitions.

You will find explanations of how appetite and metabolic rate are regulated, and I dispel some of the popular myths about metabolism. There is evidence that not all calories are equal, and that excess calories from carbohydrate or protein are less likely to be turned into body fat than calories from fat. This book discusses what is a desirable fat percentage from a health and performance point of view, and highlights the dangers of attaining a very low body fat percentage.

The latest recommendations on protein requirements for strength training are discussed and translated into practical terms. Contrary to popular belief, extra protein is not automatically converted into muscle; the fastest way to gain muscle is to achieve a slightly positive energy balance and consume the correct ratio of protein and carbohydrate. The pros and cons of protein and amino acid supplements are discussed.

Carbohydrate is the major fuel for strength training so it is essential to consume the proper amount and type of carbohydrate at the right time. This book enables you to estimate your carbohydrate and calorie needs so you can achieve high muscle glycogen levels, and maximum energy for training. Refuelling between workouts is a crucial part of the recovery process and it is important that complete refuelling is achieved in order to make rapid gains. The blood sugar raising ability of a carbohydrate is measured by its glycaemic index. Knowledge of the glycaemic index will allow you to optimise glycogen storage and blood sugar levels.

Trainers are bombarded with a vast, confusing array of nutritional supplements claiming to enhance muscle growth, mass and strength. Do growth hormone promoters work? Do plant extracts really boost testosterone production? What is the latest evidence for supplements such as creatine, glutamine and caffeine? This manual considers the scientific support for such products and will help you make an informed choice.

Exercises for each muscle group are clearly described. The step-by-step technique guide will ensure you perform them safely and gain maximum benefit. Tips and variations are given for each exercise so your programme can be infinitely varied. A unique feature of the book is a consideration of various body symmetry problems which can be corrected by a specific training programme. For example, if you have a narrow back, straight hamstrings, shapeless arms or a rounded tummy, you can re-shape that body part by following the advice in this section of the book.

The Complete Guide to Strength Training deals with those areas of nutrition relevant to strength training. These are applied in the wider context of sports nutrition in another of my books, *The Complete Guide to Sports Nutrition*, which gives practical advice on nutrition relevant to other sports.

This manual promises to speed your progress towards your fitness and nutritional goals. Whether you are just beginning a strength programme or you are an advanced trainer in search of new knowledge to inspire your training programme, this book will be invaluable. Armed with the latest scientifically-proven methods, you will reach higher levels than you imagine. I wish you every success. Train hard and eat well!

ANITA BEAN

CHAPTER 1

Why train for strength?

Within this book the term 'strength training' is used in a generic context. It refers to resistance training performed primarily to enhance a person's appearance, symmetry, strength, and well-being.

Over the last few years numerous studies have shown that strength training produces many health and fitness benefits for people of all ages and sexes. Medical bodies, fitness professionals, coaches and doctors now advocate strength training for everyone.

Here are 13 reasons to strength train.

(1) To increase muscle mass and strength

Weight training stimulates the production of new muscle proteins, namely *actin* and *myosin*, which form larger muscle fibres. Research has shown that a basic weight training programme of just 25 minutes followed for three days a week can increase muscle mass by approximately 3 lbs over an eight-week period. A well-planned weight training programme trains all muscle groups, which leads to balanced muscle development. In contrast, most endurance activities strengthen and increase endurance only in certain muscles and certain movements.

(2) To strengthen tendons and ligaments

Weight training increases joint stability by increasing the strength of the tendons and ligaments. The stress produced by strength training is also transferred to the tendons and ligaments, which increases the production of *collagen proteins*, thus causing an increase in their structural strength.

(3) To avoid age-related muscle loss

Muscle mass and strength tend to decrease with age. Without strength training, adults typically lose 5—7 lbs of muscle every decade. Muscle *atrophy* (loss) occurs primarily in the *fast twitch* muscle fibres (those involved in strength and explosive activities). Thus, strength training helps to prevent muscle and strength loss. The same cannot be said for most forms of cardiovascular exercise – only strength training maintains muscle mass and strength as we get older.

(4) To increase bone density

Women over the age of 35 lose about 1% of bone mass per year, a process that is accelerated after the menopause. Strength training improves bone strength and increases bone *osteoproteins* and mineral content. Studies show that the bones under the most stress from weight training have the highest bone mineral content. For example, it has been demonstrated that there are significant increases in the mineral content of the upper femur (thigh) after four months of strength training. An American study found that women who followed a weight training programme twice a week for one year developed 76% greater bone strength than those who did no strength training. These findings therefore suggest that weight training reduces the risk of *osteoporosis* and bone fractures.

(5) To increase metabolic rate

Strength training increases the resting metabolic rate, the energy required for tissue maintenance and essential functions. This is due to the fact that strength training increases muscle tissue which has a higher energy requirement than fat tissue, i.e. muscle tissue is metabolically active. People who strength train therefore use more calories throughout the day.

Research has shown that adding 3 lbs of muscle increases the resting metabolic rate by 7% and our daily calorie requirement by 15%. Strength training also increases exercise metabolism. At rest, 1 lb of muscle tissue requires 35 kcal per day. During exercise, energy expenditure rises dramatically, five to ten times above the resting level. Thus the more muscle tissue you have, the greater the number of calories expended during exercise and at rest.

The reduction in metabolic rate experienced by most people as they get older is due largely to loss of muscle tissue. This loss accounts for a 2—5% decrease in resting metabolic rate per decade which may translate to unwanted weight (fat) gain. Therefore, strength training is an excellent way of preserving muscle mass, preventing a reduction of metabolic rate and avoiding fat gain with age.

(6) To reduce body fat

Strength training can help reduce body fat by increasing resting metabolic rate and therefore daily calorie expenditure. A study has shown that strength training produced a loss of 4 lbs of fat after three months of training despite a 15% increase in calorie intake. Another study of 282 adult beginners found that after eight weeks of strength training and aerobic exercise, they lost almost 9 lbs of fat and gained 3 lbs of muscle; a significant improvement in body composition.

(7) To improve glucose metabolism

Strength training increases insulin sensitivity and improves glucose tolerance due to favourable changes in body composition and increases in maximal aerobic capacity. These are both important factors in preventing Type II (maturity onset) diabetes and coronary heart disease.

(8) To reduce blood pressure

Strength training has been shown to lower *systolic* and *diastolic* blood pressure. The effect is even greater if strength training is combined with aerobic training. An American study found that a combination of two months of strength training and aerobic exercise resulted in a decrease in systolic blood pressure of 5 mm Hg, and diastolic blood pressure of 3 mm Hg.

(9) To reduce blood cholesterol and blood fats

Studies have demonstrated improvements in blood cholesterol and blood *triglycerides* (fats) as a result of several weeks of strength training.

(10) To improve appearance

Personal appearance is greatly improved by strength training due to increased muscle tone, strength, function and improved posture. Changes in body composition mean an increase in lean mass and decrease in fat mass, both of which greatly enhance personal appearance.

(11) To improve posture

Strength training greatly improves overall posture as well as correcting specific posture faults. A number of factors influence our posture including skeletal structure, basic body type, strength and flexibility. Obviously, the first and second factors are controlled by our genetic make-up and cannot be altered. However, strength and flexibility can be changed through training or disuse (i.e. increased or decreased demand). Imbalances in these two components lead to posture faults, but these may be corrected through specific strength training and stretching.

(12) To reduce injuries

A well-conditioned and well-balanced musculo-skeletal system has a much smaller chance of sustaining injury. A stronger body is better able to avoid or resist impact injuries from falls and activities such as running or jumping. Muscle imbalances are a common cause of injury, for example underdeveloped hamstrings relative to the quadriceps (thigh) can make the knee joint unstable, thus increasing injury risk.

The majority of lower back problems are due to muscle weakness or imbalance. Strength training will improve the strength of the lower back muscles and other muscles involved in posture, thus reducing the likelihood of injury. A study found that patients suffering lower back pain had significantly less pain after ten weeks of specific strength exercises.

(13) To improve psychological well-being

All types of exercise help to reduce stress, anxiety and depression, and to uplift mood and increase relaxation. Weight training may help decrease muscle tension even further due to the intensity of the muscular contractions. It also improves body image which has a major effect on psychological well-being. A study at Auburn University in the U.S.A. compared the body image of powerlifters, bodybuilders, runners and sedentary students after an equal period of training. Bodybuilders and runners had a significantly better body image compared with the other groups.

The myths of weight training

Despite these well-recognised benefits of strength training, there are many myths which still exist. Here are some of the most popular misconceptions, along with the scientific facts.

Strength training makes women look too bulky

On the contrary, strength training actually enhances a woman's femininity. It improves the tone and definition of the muscles, creating a firmer and more shapely appearance. Increases in muscle mass can be made but women can never achieve the muscle bulk of men. They have much smaller amounts of the male sex hormone, *testosterone*, which is responsible for muscle building, and much higher amounts of the female sex hormone, *oestrogen*. This hormonal balance prevents the development of large or masculine looking muscles through strength training.

If you stop training muscle turns to fat

It is impossible for muscle to turn to fat as they are two completely different types of body tissue. Muscle mass and strength will gradually decrease if you stop training (some physiologists believe that a muscle will never quite return to its pre-training state), and fat stores will increase if you eat more calories than you need over a period of time. However, one will not turn into the other! Once a certain muscle mass has been achieved through regular strength training, this can be maintained by training less frequently (once or twice a week).

Weight training makes you muscle-bound and will ruin your flexibility

This is not true. Increasing your muscle mass does not make you muscle-bound, reduce your flexibility or make you lose your speed. Strength training, performed correctly, can actually improve flexibility as the muscle is exercised through its complete and natural range of movement. If flexibility is reduced it is because the individual did not train correctly, e.g. performed exercises with an incomplete range of movement or overdeveloped one muscle group (such as the quads) in relation to the opposing group (such as the hamstrings). In any case, stretching the muscle before and after training will prevent the muscle shortening and increase its flexibility. Also, it has been demonstrated that a strong muscle can contract more quickly and generate more power than a weak one. In fact, the physiques of world-class sprinters are very muscular, which goes to prove that increased muscle mass does not hinder your speed or your flexibility.

Strength training harms the joints

The opposite is true. When properly and safely performed, strength training improves the strength of the ligaments which hold a joint together, thus making it more stable and less prone to injury. Controlled, no-impact movements used in strength training place far less stress on the joints than most other forms of exercise. Impact movements such as running and jumping can unduly stress the ligaments and make the joints more susceptible to injury. Thus, strength training is a good way of strengthening the joints.

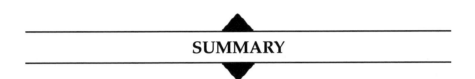

SUMMARY

- ◆ Weight training provides many health and fitness benefits.
- ◆ The fitness benefits include increases in muscle, tendon and ligament strength, in joint stability, in overall lean body mass, and in basal metabolic rate.
- ◆ The health benefits include increased bone strength and density, improved glucose metabolism, reduced blood cholesterol, and reduced blood pressure.
- ◆ Weight training can help prevent or delay the age-related decline in lean tissue mass, strength, bone density and basal metabolic rate.
- ◆ Weight training improves appearance, posture and self-esteem. It causes a favourable change in body composition, increasing muscle mass and tone and reducing body fat which, in turn, enhances body image.
- ◆ It is a myth that weight training makes a person muscle-bound, reduces flexibility, or harms the joints. Muscle does not turn to fat.
- ◆ Weight training enhances both the male and female physique; it does not produce bulky muscles in women.

Getting started

Where to train?

Whether you decide to train at home or at a gym, you should seek the advice of a professional instructor to demonstrate the exercises, at least for your initial workouts. Both home and gym environments offer different advantages and disadvantages.

At a gym

A gym can offer a greater variety of equipment including free weights, machines and cardiovascular equipment. There will also be instructors on hand to ensure that you are training correctly, offer advice and help you develop your training programme. It can be more motivating to train with other people and in a sociable club atmosphere. You may have access to other facilities such as a swimming pool, fitness classes, saunas and a cafeteria or bar.

However, membership can be expensive, although once you've paid you may be more motivated to stick to your programme and less likely to skip workouts. Overcrowding, particularly during peak times, may also be a problem.

At home

Some people prefer to train in the privacy of their own home. Training at home can be more convenient than training in a gym. It means you can train when you like and you don't have to travel to the gym, so it can save time.

However, the initial outlay for home gym equipment can be expensive, and your budget and available space will probably limit you to only the basics. Initial enthusiasm may wear off fast and, unless you set aside specific times to work out, you can always find other things to do instead. It can be difficult to motivate yourself and push yourself hard enough in a home environment to achieve significant gains.

◆ *Finding a good gym checklist* ◆

Travelling distance and time Decide how far you are prepared to travel. If the journey takes you more than 15—20 minutes you are unlikely to visit the gym regularly in the long term once the initial novelty has worn off.

Type of equipment Is there a good range of equipment to suit your needs? If you want to build mass, you will need plenty of free weights (barbells and dumbbells), benches and racks. If you are more interested in general fitness and toning, you may prefer a greater range of machines and lighter free weights.

Standard and safety of equipment Good equipment does not need to be state-of-the-art shiny machinery. Check that the equipment is well maintained with no broken or loose attachments, and is regularly cleaned and tested.

Gym layout The gym should be well ventilated and well laid out with enough space between equipment to prevent accidents and overcrowding.

Atmosphere and motivation The gym environment should be motivating for you as an individual. Some gyms are very busy and noisy, others are quieter; it is important to train in an atmosphere that suits your temperament. Try to get an idea of the type of members who train there – are they serious bodybuilders or general fitness trainers, sociable or quiet?

Instruction Check that the instructors are professionally qualified. Most instructors in the U.K. will have a certificate in fitness training or weight training, or hold a degree in sports science or a related subject. You can get advice on suitable qualifications from the Exercise Association for England or the Sports Council.

Arrange a trial workout Most gyms will be happy to arrange a trial workout. Arrange to work out at the same time as you plan to exercise so you can see whether the gym becomes overcrowded and you need to queue for equipment.

Cost Make sure you find out the true cost of joining a gym. Some require an initial non-refundable joining fee, plus an annual or monthly membership subscription. Others may allow you to pay for each workout. Multiply this by the number of times you intend to train per year. Make sure you are clear about what the membership buys you, whether you need to pay extra for other facilities, and ask about different payment methods. Find out whether any discounts are available (e.g. off-peak membership).

Getting motivated

(1) Set clear goals
Your goals should be S.M.A.R.T.

Specific Write down exactly how much lean weight you wish to gain or how much fat you wish to lose; your desired body measurements; how much weight you wish to lift on exercises such as the bench press, squat and dead lift.

Measurable In terms of body weight, body measurements or weight lifted.

Agreed Discuss and agree your goals with someone – a qualified instructor, your partner, a friend.

Realistic The goals should be attainable for your body size, natural shape (*see* page 17) and weight.

Time-scaled Set a clear time scale for reaching your goals; set mini goals which can be reached every month and long-term goals which can be reached in a year.

(2) Have a realistic role model
Role models can help to motivate you and give you a good mental picture of what you will look like. Pick one with a similar natural body type, shape and size as you – that way, you know you can achieve your goals and won't lose heart if you don't look like your role model after a period of training. Don't think you can look exactly like Arnold Schwarzenegger if you are naturally very slim, or Claudia Schiffer if you are naturally short and stocky.

(3) Make training fun
Training should be enjoyable; it should give you a buzz and make you feel good about yourself. If you have to force yourself to work out when you really don't enjoy it, you will not train hard enough to make sufficient gains, and you are more likely to give up. Many people who train for years without enjoying it stay the same size and fail to get any stronger. So make sure you choose the right training environment and the right training programme. That way, training will become part of your lifestyle.

(4) Work out with a partner
Training with someone else will increase your motivation, make training more fun, allow you to train harder and so achieve faster gains, decrease the chances of you skipping workouts, and help you

to stick to your training programme. Choose someone with similar goals to your own but not necessarily the same ability. The important thing is that you can motivate each other.

(5) Keep a training diary
Keep a training diary to record your progress. You can write down details of each exercise, set and how much weight you used; how you felt before and after each workout; what and how much you ate each day; details of any other exercise you took; your body measurements.

(6) Maintain variety
Change your workout every six sessions initially and then every four to six weeks, to keep boredom at bay and increase the likelihood of continual improvement. When you start a strength training programme, gains are rapid (strength increases by up to 72% in the first four weeks) but then slow down or reach a plateau. If you follow the same workout week after week you will soon lose interest, your workout intensity will drop, training gains will slow down and you will give up. Change the split of your programme (*see* page 44); the order of exercises; the type of exercises; the weights used (*see* page 43). Take a complete rest from weight training every few months and spend a week or two doing a completely different activity.

(7) Use a personal trainer
If you do not have a training partner or you need extra motivation, consider using a personal trainer either on an occasional or regular basis. A personal trainer will not only design your programme but will help keep you motivated. He or she will make sure that you are on track with your goals and that you don't skip your workout, give you advice, help you get far more out of your workout, and also allow you to train at a time that is convenient for you.

(8) Reward yourself
Give yourself rewards when you have reached a mini goal, for example, a new training outfit, a trip to the theatre, a meal out, new clothes, a sports massage appointment, whatever gives you something to look forward to.

Workout accessories

Training belt

A training belt is advantageous for exercises which place considerable stress on the vertebrae, such as heavy squats, dead lifts and shoulder presses. It helps to provide extra support for the lower back by increasing the abdominal wall pressure. The tighter the belt, the greater the abdominal pressure against the spine, which thereby helps to support the back and keeps your torso firmer.

Do not rely on a belt for lighter exercises or if you have a lower back injury or weakness. Using a belt for any other exercises in your workout can lead to a weakening of the abdominal muscles. Therefore, use a belt only when lifting heavy weights which would otherwise place stress on the lower back.

Training gloves

Training gloves give your palms just enough padding to improve your grip of the bar or dumbbells and prevent calluses and blisters forming on your hands. They are useful for any pressing, pulling or curling movement.

Using gloves is also more hygienic than using bare hands – weight training apparatus can be sweaty and dirty, and an ideal breeding place for germs. However, do make sure you regularly wash your gloves.

Straps

Grip failure can be a limiting factor in pulling movements such as chins, rowing and lat pulldowns. Up to a point, training without straps will help to develop the forearm muscles and strengthen your grip. However, once your grip strength starts to limit the amount of weight you can use or reduce the number of reps you can do, you should use straps. They will help you to focus on the muscle you are training and reduce the involvement of limiting muscles such as forearms.

Straps are therefore advantageous for most back exercises such as dead lifts, chins, lat pulldowns, seated rows, one-arm dumbbell rows, and shrugs.

Knee wraps

Knee wraps can help support the knee joint during heavy leg exercises such as dead lifts and squats. They help to stabilise the joint by assisting the ligaments. As with training belts, do not rely on wraps if you have a knee injury or to help you lift heavier weights than your strength allows. They are best used for maximal weights (e.g. twice your body weight) rather than as a crutch for lighter sets.

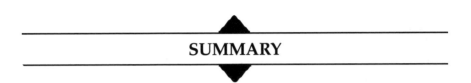

SUMMARY

- The benefits of training in a commercial gym include access to a wider range of equipment, professional instruction, motivation and social contact.
- A home gym offers greater privacy and convenience but the equipment can be limited and, initially, expensive.
- Motivation is a fundamental part of a training programme. Trainers should set clear, specific and realistic goals.
- Motivation can be increased by choosing a role model, training with a partner, making the workout varied and fun, keeping a training diary, rewarding your progress and using a personal trainer.
- Workout accessories such as training belts, gloves, straps and knee wraps can assist your progress when used under appropriate conditions.

3

Re-shaping your body

The basic shape of your body is determined by your genetic make-up and your hormonal balance. The width of your shoulders, the size of your hips, the length of your limbs, and the relative proportions of various parts of your body are all dependent on your natural body type and shape. The basic body proportions and musculo-skeletal structure for each body type and shape are very similar – you can be tall or short yet still share the same body type. Your genes also dictate how readily you store fat and where it is distributed.

Although you cannot change your genetic body type, by combining the right type of weight training and aerobic programme with a carefully planned nutrition programme you can improve your shape. Some body types respond to exercise and diet more readily than others, for example, when *android* (apple-shaped) individuals lose weight this is mostly from the abdominal region, thus creating a very different shape. When *gynaecoid* (pear-shaped) individuals lose weight they tend to do so evenly from all over the body thus creating a smaller version of the same shape.

Four of the most common body types are described below together with re-shaping strategies. Find the type that most resembles your shape. (*See* fig. 1, on page 17.)

The 'android' or 'apple' shape

Your natural shape is characterised by a small, narrow pelvis, broad shoulders and fairly muscular limbs. Your torso tends to be broad and straight, and with your narrow hips gives the appearance of being thick-waisted. This is the most common body type in men (due to the influence of the male sex hormones, such as testosterone) but can occur in women too. Apple-shaped women have relatively high

Figure 1 *The four most common body types.*

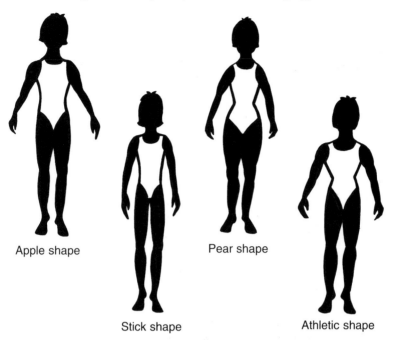

Apple shape   Pear shape

Stick shape   Athletic shape

levels of male sex hormones and so tend to have a fairly masculine shape which makes them well-suited to sports requiring strength.

Fat tends to be stored mainly in the upper torso, accentuating the thick-waisted appearance or, if fat gain is substantial, creating handlebars at the sides of the waist or the classic 'pot belly'. Despite this, the hips, legs and arms remain slim and muscular. Fat is also stored intra-abdominally, that is in the deeper layers close to the internal organs. This increases the risk of metabolic disorders such as high blood cholesterol, high blood pressure, diabetes and heart disease (due to the close proximity of the fat tissue to the liver).

Re-shape strategy

♦ Reduce waist size by reducing excess fat from the abdominal region. You cannot spot reduce fat, however. In this case, fat will be lost from all areas of the body but the shape change will be especially noticeable around the abdomen.
♦ Improve appearance of mid-section by increasing the tone and strength of the abdominal muscles.
♦ Strengthen upper and lower body equally.

17

Weight training programme

Stage 1 (0—1 month)   General circuit weight training programme for beginners. Follow this stage if you have not trained with weights before.

Select a suitable weight that will allow you to complete the chosen number of reps with relative ease. You should feel fairly breathless but your muscles should not 'burn' or reach the point of failure.

Take 10—20 seconds rest between each exercise.

Sample circuit weight training programme

Squat	15 reps
Curl up	15 reps
Bench press	15 reps
Leg extension	15 reps
Reverse curl up	15 reps
Shoulder press (dumbbells)	15 reps
Lying leg curl	15 reps
The crunch	15 reps
Leg press	15 reps
Biceps curl	15 reps
Oblique curl up	15 reps
Lat pulldown	15 reps
Triceps pushdown	15 reps
Upright row	15 reps
Repeat circuit 2—3 times	

Stage 2 (1—6 months)   Two-way split for intermediate trainers. Repeat each workout twice a week, so that you train four days per week, e.g. Monday, Tuesday; repeated Thursday, Friday.

Stage 3 (6 months +)   Four-way split training programme for advanced trainers. Perform each workout once a week so you complete a total of four workouts per week, e.g. Monday, Tuesday, Thursday, Saturday.

Two-way split training programme

Day 1		Day 2	
Leg press or squat	3 x 12	Shoulder press	3 x 12
Leg extension	2 x 10	Upright row	3 x 10
Leg curl	2 x 10	Lat pulldown behind neck	3 x 12
Bench press	3 x 12	One-arm dumbbell row	3 x 10
Incline flye	3 x 10	Triceps extension	4 x 10
Barbell curl	4 x 10	Curl up	2 x 20
The crunch	2 x 20	Lying side bend	2 x 20
Oblique crunch	2 x 20	The flattener	2 x 20
Reverse curl	2 x 20		

Four-way split training programme

Day 1	Day 2	Day 3	Day 4
Bench press 3 x 8—10	Lat pulldown 3x 8—10	Squat 4 x 8—15	Shoulder press 3 x 8—10
Incline dumbbell press 3 x 8—10	Seated row 3 x 8—10	Lunge 4 x 10—12	Lateral raise 3 x 8—10
Flye or pullover 3 x 8—10	Close grip pulldown 3 x 8—10	Leg curl 4 x 8—12	Upright row 3 x 8—10
Barbell curl 3 x 8—12	Curl up/crunch 2 x 20	Calf raise 6 x 12—15	Triceps dip 3 x 8—12
Concentration curl 3 x 8—12	Hanging leg raise 2 x 20	The crunch 2 x 20	Triceps pushdown 3 x 8—12
The crunch 2 x 20	Lying side bend 2 x 20	Reverse crunch 2 x 20	Hanging leg raise 2 x 20
Reverse crunch 2 x 20		Oblique crunch 2 x 20	Lying side bend 2 x 20
Oblique crunch 2 x 20			

Aerobic programme

Choose one or more of the following activities:

- fitness walking (4 mph)
- step aerobics/stepping machine
- swimming
- cycling
- aerobics class
- jogging
- rowing machine.

Week 1	3 sessions 15—20 minutes
Week 2	3 sessions 20—30 minutes
Week 3	3—4 sessions 30 minutes
Week 4	4 sessions 35—40 minutes
Week 5	4—5 sessions 40 minutes
Week 6	5 sessions 40—45 minutes
Week 7 onwards	5 sessions 45 minutes

The 'gynaecoid' or 'pear' shape

The gynaecoid shape is characterised by the classic pear shape. Your shoulders are narrower than your hips, you have a naturally small waist and narrow upper back and your arms and legs are relatively slim. This is the most common body type in women (due to high levels of the female sex hormones) although it can occur in men as well.

You tend to store fat readily, mainly around the hips, thighs and the back of the upper arms, thus accentuating the pear shape. However, the forearms and shins remain slim. The fat is mostly *subcutaneous*, that is it is located immediately below the skin so it is more visible to the eye and feels softer to the touch. It is sometimes called *cellulite* when it has a distinctive lumpy 'orange peel' appearance. This is not a special kind of fat; its outward appearance is due to the criss-crossing of connective tissue fibres in the fat tissue beneath the skin.

Re-shape strategy

- Reduce pear shape; create more of an 'X' shape by building muscle mass in the upper body.
- Increase (muscular) width of shoulders and upper back to balance hips.
- Tone/strengthen thighs and hips.

◆ Reduce excess fat from hips and thighs. Again, you cannot spot reduce fat. Fat will be lost from all areas of the body, but more noticeably from the hips and thighs.

Weight training programme

Stage 1 (0—1 month)   General circuit weight training programme for beginners. Follow this stage if you have not trained with weights before.

Select a suitable weight that will allow you to complete the chosen number of reps with relative ease. You should feel fairly breathless but your muscles should not 'burn' or reach the point of failure.

Take 10—20 seconds rest between each exercise.

Sample circuit weight training programme

Lat pulldown	15 reps
Lateral raise	15 reps
Shoulder press	15 reps
Leg extension	15 reps
Leg curl	15 reps
Oblique curl up	15 reps
The crunch	15 reps
Pec deck	15 reps
Biceps curl	15 reps
Triceps pushdown	15 reps
Seated row	15 reps
Upright row	15 reps
Repeat circuit 2—3 times	

Stage 2 (1—6 months)   Two-way split for intermediate trainers. Repeat each workout twice a week, so that you train four days per week, e.g. Monday, Tuesday; repeated Thursday, Friday.

Stage 3 (6 months +)   Four-way split training programme for advanced trainers. Perform each workout once a week so you complete a total of four workouts per week, e.g. Monday, Tuesday, Thursday, Saturday.

Two-way split training programme

Day 1		Day 2	
Squat	3 x 15	Bench press	3 x 8
Rear lunge	2 x 15	Incline flye	3 x 8
Shoulder press	3 x 8	Lat pulldown	3 x 8
Lateral raise	3 x 8	Seated row	3 x 8
Upright row	3 x 8	Dumbbell curl	3 x 10
The crunch	1 x 20	Triceps extension	3 x 10
Oblique crunch	1 x 20		
Reverse curl	1 x 20		

Four-way split training programme

Day 1	Day 2	Day 3	Day 4
Incline bench press 3 x 8	Squat 3 x 15	Lateral dumbbell raise 3 x 8	Chins 3 x 8
Dumbbell press 3 x 8	Rear lunge 3 x 15	Dumbbell press 3 x 8	One-arm dumbbell row 3 x 8
Incline flye 3 x 8	Leg extension 3 x 15	Upright row 3 x 8	Lat pulldown behind neck 3 x 8
Barbell curl 4 x 8	Calf raise 6 x 12—15	Triceps extension 4 x 8	Hanging leg raise 2 x 20
	The crunch 2 x 20		Lying side bend 2 x 20
	Oblique crunch 2 x 20		
	Reverse cunch 2 x 8		

Aerobic programme

Choose one or more of the following activities:

◆ fitness walking (4 mph)
◆ step aerobics/stepping machine
◆ swimming
◆ cycling
◆ aerobics class
◆ jogging
◆ rowing machine.

Week 1	3 sessions 15—20 minutes
Week 2	3 sessions 20—30 minutes
Week 3	3—4 sessions 30 minutes
Week 4	4 sessions 35—40 minutes
Week 5	4—5 sessions 40 minutes
Week 6	5 sessions 40—45 minutes
Week 7 onwards	5 sessions 45 minutes

The 'stick' shape

The natural 'stick' shape is characterised by a straight, streamlined torso. The shoulders are narrow and about the same width as the hips, and the legs and arms are long and slim. Stick-shaped people have a rather boyish shape lacking in classic curves. Tall stick-shaped women can look willowy (the classic model shape) and stick-shaped men tend to look rangy.

You do not put weight on readily but if excess fat occurs it tends to be stored evenly around the abdomen. Thus stick-shaped individuals seldom have a weight problem and are often the envy of plumper friends.

Re-shape strategy

◆ Increase overall muscle mass.
◆ Build upper and lower body equally to give more shape.
◆ Increase overall strength.
◆ Maintain low body fat.

Weight training programme

Stage 1 (0—1 month) General circuit weight training programme for beginners. Follow this stage if you have not trained with weights before.

23

Select a suitable weight that will allow you to complete the chosen number of reps with relative ease. You should feel fairly breathless but your muscles should not 'burn' or reach the point of failure.

Take 10—20 seconds rest between each exercise.

Sample circuit weight training programme

Squat	15 reps
Bench press	15 reps
Leg extension	15 reps
Shoulder press (dumbbells)	15 reps
The crunch	15 reps
Lat pulldown	15 reps
Lying leg curl	15 reps
Biceps curl	15 reps
Oblique curl up	15 reps
Triceps pushdown	15 reps
Leg press	15 reps
Upright row	15 reps
Repeat circuit 2—3 times	

Stage 2 (1—6 months) Two-way split for intermediate trainers. Repeat each workout twice a week, so that you train four days per week, e.g. Monday, Tuesday; repeated Thursday, Friday.

Two-way split training programme

Day 1		Day 2	
Dead lift	4 x 10	Shoulder press	4 x 10
Leg press or squat	4 x 10	Upright row	4 x 10
Bench press	4 x 10	Lat pulldown	4 x 10
Incline dumbbell press	4 x 10	Seated row	4 x 10
Barbell curl	4 x 10	Triceps pushdown	4 x 10
		The crunch	2 x 20
		Oblique crunch	2 x 20

Stage 3 (6 months +) Four-way split training programme for advanced trainers. Perform each workout once a week so you complete a total of four workouts per week, e.g. Monday, Tuesday, Thursday, Saturday.

Four-way split training programme

Day 1	Day 2	Day 3	Day 4
Squat 4 x 6—10	Bench press 4 x 8	Chins 3 x 8	Shoulder press 4 x 8—10
Dead lift 4 x 6—10	Incline dumbbell press 4 x 8	One-arm dumbbell row 3 x 8	Lateral raise or upright row 4 x 8
Leg extension 4 x 6—10	Barbell curl or preacher curl 4 x 8	Close grip pulldown 3 x 8	Triceps extension 3 x 8
Leg curl 4 x 8—12	The crunch 2 x 20		The crunch 2 x 20
Calf raise 4 x 10—15	Oblique crunch 2 x 20		Hanging leg raise 2 x 20
	Reverse crunch 2 x 20		

Aerobic programme

Choose one or more of the following activities:

♦ fitness walking (4 mph)
♦ step aerobics/stepping machine
♦ swimming
♦ cycling
♦ aerobics class
♦ jogging
♦ rowing machine.

Week 1	2 sessions 15—20 minutes
Week 2	3 sessions 20—30 minutes
Week 3	3 sessions 20—30 minutes
Week 4	3 sessions 20—40 minutes
Week 5	3 sessions 20—45 minutes
Week 6	3 sessions 20—45 minutes
Week 7 onwards	3 sessions 20—45 minutes

The 'athletic' shape

The athletic shape has relatively broad shoulders, a narrow waist and narrow hips. Your shoulders are wider than your hips, creating a classic 'V' taper, while your torso and limbs are well muscled. An athletic build is particularly well-suited to sports requiring strength, speed, agility and power, as well as aesthetic sports such as bodybuilding.

With training, you gain muscle mass more readily than other body types, thus accentuating your natural 'V' taper. You do not tend to store fat readily, however if excess weight gain does occur, it tends to be evenly distributed over the body or just around the abdomen.

Re-shape strategy

◆ Increase overall muscle mass and strength.
◆ Build upper and lower body equally to maintain athletic shape.
◆ Maintain low body fat.

Weight training programme

Stage 1 (0—1 month) General circuit weight training programme for beginners. Follow this stage if you have not trained with weights before.

Sample circuit weight training programme

Squat	15 reps
Bench press	15 reps
Leg extension	15 reps
Shoulder press (dumbbells)	15 reps
The crunch	15 reps
Lat pulldown	15 reps
Lying leg curl	15 reps
Biceps curl	15 reps
Oblique curl up	15 reps
Triceps pushdown	15 reps
Leg press	15 reps
Upright row	15 reps
Repeat circuit 2—3 times	

Select a suitable weight that will allow you to complete the chosen number of reps with relative ease. You should feel fairly breathless but your muscles should not 'burn' or reach the point of failure.

Take 10—20 seconds rest between each exercise.

Two-way split training programme

Day 1		Day 2	
Dead lift	4 x 10	Lat pulldown	4 x 10
Leg press or squat	4 x 10	Seated row	4 x 10
Shoulder press	4 x 10	Bench press	4 x 10
Upright row	4 x 10	Incline dumbbell press	4 x 10
Triceps extension	4 x 10	Barbell curl	4 x 10
		The crunch	2 x 20
		Oblique crunch	2 x 20

Stage 2 (1—6 months) Two-way split for intermediate trainers. Repeat each workout twice a week, so that you train four days per week, e.g. Monday, Tuesday; repeated Thursday, Friday.

Four-way split training programme

Day 1	Day 2	Day 3	Day 4
Dead lift 4 x 10	Bench press 3 x 10	Chins 3 x 10	Shoulder press 3 x 10
Squat or leg press 4 x 10	Flye 3 x 10	Seated row 3 x 10	Upright row 3 x 10
Leg extension 4 x 6—10	Incline dumbbell press or flye 3 x 10	Close grip chin or pulldown 3 x 8	Lateral raise 3 x 10
Leg curl 4 x 8—12	Barbell curl 3 x 10	The crunch 2 x 20	Triceps extension 3 x 8
Calf raise 4 x 10—15	Dumbbell curl 3 x 10	Oblique crunch 2 x 20	Triceps pushdown 3 x 8
The crunch 2 x 20		Reverse crunch 2 x 20	
Hanging leg raise 2 x 20			

Stage 3 (6 months +) Four-way split training programme for advanced trainers. Perform each workout once a week so you complete a total of four workouts per week, e.g. Monday, Tuesday, Thursday, Saturday.

Aerobic programme

Choose one or more of the following activities:

- fitness walking (4 mph)
- step aerobics/stepping machine
- swimming
- cycling
- aerobics class
- jogging
- rowing machine.

Week 1	2 sessions 15—20 minutes
Week 2	3 sessions 20—30 minutes
Week 3	3 sessions 20—30 minutes
Week 4	3 sessions 20—40 minutes
Week 5	3—4 sessions 20—45 minutes
Week 6	3—4 sessions 20—45 minutes
Week 7 onwards	3—4 sessions 20—45 minutes

◆ *Sheldon body types* ◆

The Sheldon system classifies body types into three basic categories.

Ectomorphs have a naturally slim build with long lean limbs and narrow shoulders and hips. They have relatively little muscle bulk and don't tend to gain muscle or fat easily.

Mesomorphs have a naturally athletic build with wide shoulders and narrow hips. They tend to have thick bones and gain muscle readily.

Endomorphs have a naturally stocky, rounded build with wide shoulders and wide hips. They tend to have an even distribution of fat and gain both fat and muscle readily.

In practice, most people are a mixture of these three body types and can score points out of ten for the characteristics they possess of each type. For example, you may share most of the characteristics of a mesomorph (wide shoulders, narrow hips) but have a small tendency towards an endomorph (gain fat readily). Thus you may score 2/10; 8/10; 4/10 for ecto-, meso- and endomorph characteristics respectively.

Figure 2 Sheldon body types. *Mesomorph* (LEFT); *Endomorph* (CENTRE); *Ectomorph* (RIGHT)

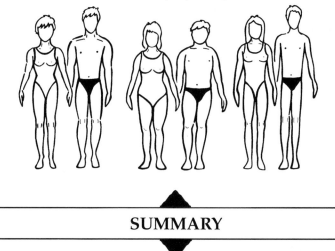

SUMMARY

- The basic shape of your body is determined by your genetic make-up and your hormonal balance.
- It is possible to categorise your body shape into one of four types: the android/apple shape, the gynaecoid/pear shape, the stick shape or the athletic shape.
- You can improve or re-balance your shape through a specific weight training, aerobic and nutrition programme.
- The android shape is characterised by narrow hips, a thick waist, slim limbs and a tendency to store fat around the abdomen. This shape can be improved by building upper and lower body mass, reducing excess fat and toning the abdominal muscles.
- The gynaecoid shape is characterised by narrow shoulders and a lean upper body, wide hips and a tendency to store fat around the hips and thighs. This shape can be re-balanced by increasing upper body mass, toning the hips and thighs and reducing excess fat.
- The stick shape is characterised by a thin, streamlined torso, long, slim limbs, small muscles and a low body fat percentage. This shape can be improved by increasing overall muscle mass and developing both upper and lower body.
- The athletic shape is characterised by broad shoulders, a narrow waist and hips and a 'V'-shaped torso. This shape can be enhanced by a balanced weight training programme and by maintaining low body fat stores.

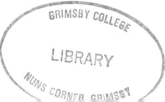

All about muscles

This chapter will help you gain a greater understanding of why and how your muscles respond to weight training. It explains the principles of muscle growth and strength development, knowledge you can then apply to your training programme. Some people appear to be naturally stronger than others and respond faster to a weight training programme. This is largely due to genetics, body type and hormonal balance. Your genetic make-up determines the proportion and distribution of the different types of muscle fibres you possess which, in turn, will greatly influence your ability to develop muscle mass and strength. This chapter explains how your physical performance is affected and how training can change the characteristics of some of these fibres.

How do muscles become stronger?

When muscles are worked harder than normal they will be forced to do extra work to overcome the load. This process is called overloading and leads to increases in strength through the following process.

When the muscle contracts against a resistance it stimulates a breakdown of muscle proteins and the formation of very small (micro) tears in the muscle fibres and connective tissue. This occurs primarily during the *eccentric* phase of the motion (*see* page 46). After a period of rest and recovery, new proteins are built up, the connective tissue is repaired, the muscle fibres enlarge and the muscle increases in diameter and strength.

This is not due to an increase in the number of muscle fibres (which remains the same) but to an increase in the size of filaments in the fibres. Thus each fibre becomes denser, and the denser the fibres, the more force they can generate against a resistance. In other words, the greater the size of the muscle and the density of the fibres within it, the stronger the muscle.

In addition, regular training causes an increase in the number of blood vessels in the muscle (capillarisation). This means that more oxygen, fuel and nutrients can be delivered to the muscles and metabolic waste products can be removed more readily. The overall result is one of increased efficiency, strength and size.

The attached tendons, ligaments and bones also increase in strength and so the whole surrounding structural framework becomes stronger.

The nerve pathways serving the muscle improve, allowing the muscle fibres to be used more efficiently at any one time. This accounts for the relatively rapid improvements in strength when beginning a training programme. Muscle size remains the same initially as the muscle is able to lift the weight more efficiently and so strength improves. Later, the muscle fibres enlarge and so muscle mass increases.

◆ *Muscle terms* ◆

Hypertrophy – an increase in size of the muscle cell (or fibre).

Hyperplasia – an increase in the number of cells (or fibres).

Anabolic – synthesis of complex substances from more simple ones; the building of muscle tissue; a net increase in muscle protein.

Catabolic – destructive metabolic process involving breakdown of complex materials into simpler ones; breakdown of muscle tissue; a net decrease in muscle protein.

Concentric – shortening of a muscle during contraction.

Eccentric – lengthening of a muscle under tension.

Ligament – tough connective tissue which attaches two bones to form a joint.

Tendon – the tough tissue connecting muscle to bone.

What is the difference between muscle strength and endurance?

Muscle strength is the amount of force a muscle can produce, for example the amount of weight that can be lifted. The greater the size of a muscle the greater the strength. Strength is acquired through progressive resistance training, that is, lifting heavier and heavier weights over a period of time.

Muscle endurance is the ability of a muscle to continue contracting against a resistance. This is developed by maintaining a constant workload for increasing periods of time – lifting a weight for 12 or more repetitions then building up to say 15, 20 and so on as endurance improves. Long distance cycling will develop muscle endurance in the thigh muscles, for example.

Strength training will develop both muscle strength and endurance, but the amount of weight lifted and the number of repetitions will determine which aspect is developed most. In general, using heavy weights for lower repetitions (less than 12) develops strength; using lighter weights for more repetitions develops endurance.

Are some people's muscles naturally stronger than others?

Some people seem to be able to produce great gains in muscle mass and strength. Others see only small, slow increases despite years of hard workouts, yet may be able to keep up long periods of aerobic activity with apparent ease. This is, in part, due to differences in the mix of muscle fibre types, which have an important effect on the type of activity your body is best suited to (e.g. aerobic or anaerobic). Your particular distribution of fibre types influence your strength and endurance.

Muscle fibres

There are three main types of muscle fibre:

◆ slow twitch fibres (ST)
◆ fast twitch a fibres (FTa)
◆ fast twitch b fibres (FTb).

ST fibres contract relatively slowly. They have a high endurance capacity, do not tire easily and are used mainly in low-intensity, long-duration aerobic activities such as jogging. They have many capillaries and mitochondria (the power houses of cells) and can easily make use of both fat and carbohydrate for fuel.

FT fibres in general are better suited to anaerobic activities than ST fibres and have relatively poor endurance. FTa fibres can produce more force than ST fibres but tire more easily. They have a lower endurance capacity and are used mainly during high-intensity activities such as a 1500-metre run.

The FTb fibres are similar to FTa fibres but have a poor blood supply and few mitochondria. They tire very quickly and are mainly used for explosive power activities such as sprinting and jumping. They have the highest anaerobic capacity but the lowest endurance capacity.

How does fibre type affect your performance?

On average, most muscles are composed roughly of 50% ST, 25% FTa and 25% FTb fibres, although the exact percentage varies between different muscles. Generally, a person's leg and arm muscles have similar fibre compositions, however, there are one or two exceptions. In most people, for example, the soleus muscle (lower calf) is almost entirely composed of ST fibres, whereas the deltoid muscles (shoulders) are comprised of a high proportion of FT fibres.

The proportion of different fibre types in your muscles dictates whether you are naturally suited to endurance, power or strength sports. If you have a high proportion of ST fibres (particularly in your leg muscles) you will be well-suited to endurance activities. If you have a higher proportion of FT fibres you are more likely to do well at sports involving power, sprints and strength.

Studies of élite athletes have revealed that distance runners have a significantly higher percentage of ST fibres (69—79%) in the gastrocnemius (calf muscle) compared with sprinters (24—27%), while world-class marathon runners have been reported to possess up to 99% ST fibres in their gastrocnemius. Weightlifters have a higher percentage of FT fibres (56%) in the gastrocnemius compared with distance runners (21—31%).

People with a high proportion of ST fibres will develop strength less readily than those with more FT fibres. However, it is not necessarily a straightforward relationship since there are other variables affecting strength and endurance, such as quality of training. Someone with a high proportion of ST fibres can still be stronger than someone with a high proportion of FT fibres if they have plenty of motivation and follow the correct training and nutrition programme. Your ability to reach your full potential is dependent on your mental attitude, training and diet.

Can you train the different muscle fibres?

Studies show that the distribution of the different fibre types is largely genetically determined. In fact, whether a muscle fibre becomes fast or slow twitch is determined before birth and in the first few years of life. After this time, there is little you can do to change the numbers of FT and ST fibres, although as you age you tend to lose FT fibres.

It is possible to change the function of the muscle fibre types, however, through specific kinds of training. With aerobic training, FTa fibres can learn to use more oxygen and so assume some of the characteristics of ST fibres, i.e. they become more aerobic, while FTb fibres begin to assume some of the characteristics of FTa fibres and gain greater endurance. So, endurance training does not change the fibre type but will increase the muscles' aerobic capacity. Strength training improves muscle strength and anaerobic capacity but will not change aerobic capacity.

There is evidence that heavy weight training can convert some FTb fibres into FTa fibres. Research also suggests that, with age, muscles become smaller because of loss of fibres, in particular FT fibres. However, loss of muscle size is not inevitable. Endurance and resistance training can help maintain the size of the ST and FT fibres respectively.

SUMMARY

◆ Muscles increase in strength and mass when they are subjected to overload. This is achieved by progressive resistance training.

◆ An increase in muscle size is due to an increase in muscle fibre size and density rather than an increase in the number of fibres.

◆ Strength is proportional to muscle size and is a measure of the amount of force a muscle can generate. It is developed using heavy weights and a low repetition range (6—12).

◆ Muscle endurance is the ability of a muscle to continue contracting against a resistance. It is developed using light or moderate weights and a higher repetition range (more than 12).

◆ The proportion of fast and slow twitch muscle fibres influences your ability to develop strength, mass and endurance.

◆ Slow twitch fibres are well suited to endurance activities; FTa fibres have many mitochondria and are suited to explosive power activities; FTb fibres are similar to FTa fibres but have fewer mitochondria and tire more quickly.

◆ Individuals with a high percentage of FT fibres develop mass and strength more readily. Those with a high percentage of ST fibres tend to develop strength and muscle mass more slowly.

◆ The proportion of fibre types cannot be changed although heavy weight training can cause some conversion of FTb fibres to FTa fibres.

Training methods

A major aim of any weight training programme is to continually improve muscle mass, shape and strength. When you begin weight training, gains are relatively rapid but soon slow down as the muscles adapt to the training load. To encourage the muscles to continue to hypertrophy, you must use progressive resistance training methods. That is, you must subject the muscles to a progressively greater overload. Training intensity can be increased by using a variety of techniques, detailed in this chapter.

What is overload training?

Overload training is a method of progressively working your muscles harder and harder in order to induce hypertrophy. To continue gaining strength and mass you have to increase the amount of overload. The most fundamental way of achieving overload is by increasing the resistance you place on the muscle group in one of the following ways:

◆ increasing the weight but doing the same number of repetitions
◆ increasing the repetitions or sets but keeping the weight the same
◆ reducing the time intervals between sets.

A combination of two or more of these methods can be used to achieve overload. For example, when performing the shoulder press you may be able to complete 3 sets of 8 reps with 50 kg before reaching failure. On your next workout, aim to complete 9—10 reps with that same weight, and as you get stronger increase the number of reps again.

Once you can do 12 reps, increase the weight by approximately 5% (say, to 52.5 kg). You will have to reduce the number of repetitions, perhaps to around 8 reps. Always aim to train to the point of failure, i.e. the point at which you cannot complete another rep in strict style. For variety, you can slightly reduce the rest period between sets (say from 90 seconds to 70 seconds – a minimum of 45 seconds is usually recommended). You can continue to overload your muscles by increasing the reps and weight in this manner.

How long should you leave between workouts

To increase muscle mass and strength, two key factors are required:

◆ workouts to stimulate muscle growth
◆ rest periods between workouts.

The amount of time it takes to recover between workouts depends on a number of key factors, including:

◆ the intensity of your training
◆ the duration of your training
◆ your training experience and fitness level
◆ your diet.

If you don't give your body adequate rest between workouts, you will not experience sufficient gains in mass or strength. It is only after completion of the recovery process that the muscles can grow and strengthen. Immediately after a workout the body is in a *catabolic* state. In fact, during the initial recovery period the body is basically compensating for the damage caused by the workout, replacing the damaged proteins and repairing the damaged muscles. It is during the final stages of the recovery period that growth or overcompensation takes place as the body makes sure it can better survive a similar stress in the future.

This can only take place, however, after the basic compensation phase is complete. If you attempt to train your muscles before the process is complete then you will experience only minimal growth or none at all. In other words, training before you have fully recovered is counterproductive.

It is a myth that atrophy or loss of strength begins within 72 hours of a workout. Since it may take several days for compensation to occur, it would not be possible for decompensation to begin in this short time. For this reason, many scientists now recommend experienced trainers exercise each muscle group once every 6—7 days or even less frequently. Indeed, many trainers have experienced dramatic increases in growth using this method.

How do you know if your muscles have recovered?

There is no easy and accurate way of predicting your recovery rate between workouts. In the laboratory, scientists can measure blood levels of muscle metabolites such as 3 methyl histidine and creatine phosphokinase but this is clearly not a practical measure for everyday training! Instead, a certain amount of guesswork is required. When your muscles have regained their pre-workout capacity, measured by testing your strength, you have probably recovered. There is a good deal of trial and error involved as you have to judge the 'feel' of your muscles. Obviously, if your muscles still feel sore, stiff or weak, then they have not recovered. If you find yourself stronger and able to work out harder, then you know your muscles have fully recovered. Recovery rates are also dependent on the individual – on age, nutritional status, training status, sleep, hormonal and physiological factors; you have to learn to gauge your own recovery time.

Free weights or machines?

A number of studies have indicated that free weights build strength and mass more efficiently than machines. The advantages and disadvantages of each are considered below.

(1) Balance and skill
Lifting free weights develops greater balance and motor skills than using machines. More muscle fibres and nerve inputs (motor units) are activated to balance the weight throughout the range of movement. Accessory muscles are also developed as they must work synergistically with the prime movers.

Since machines lock you into a fixed plane of movement, they reduce the contribution of accessory muscles and so require less balance and skill to perform an exercise. This may be advantageous for beginners with poor motor skills and poor muscle/posture awareness.

(2) Biomechanics

Free weights accommodate the natural leverage of the body and the changes in force generated through the range of motion. Cam machines, on the other hand, often place an increasing load on the muscle as it contracts. The theory behind such a design is that a muscle becomes stronger as it contracts, however this is not true. The fact is that muscles are not in their strongest position when they are fully contracted. Firstly, the actin and myosin filaments are crossed in this position, and therefore all the muscle fibres cannot be recruited; secondly, the parallel elastic components (the elements of the muscle that assist in the development of strength) are not in an optimal position for maximum force production.

For example, when performing a biceps curl, maximum force can be generated at the point where the forearm is parallel to the ground and this diminishes as the biceps continue to contract. However, most machines place increasing resistance on the muscle in this portion of the motion and so a lower weight has to be selected in order to complete the movement. In other words, the muscle will not receive maximum stimulus in its biomechanically favourable position. Result: slower gains in strength and size.

(3) Leverage

Another problem with machines is that they do not accommodate the natural leverage of the body. Everyone has a unique set of levers which will not exactly fit a machine. The resistance cams are set to match the strength curves of the average person, which means that for everyone else the heaviest resistance occurs at inappropriate angles. Thus, a lighter weight has to be selected in order to complete the motion, reducing the intensity of the exercise and the training effect.

(4) Plane of movement

Machines require the limbs to move in a fixed plane which will not develop co-ordination skills. It also reduces the stimulus received by the muscles and so strength and size gains will be smaller.

Barbells and dumbbells allow the limbs to move in their natural arcs. This helps develop greater co-ordination skills and facilitates greater strength development.

(5) Variability

Several different variations of the same exercise may be performed with free weights, for example bench presses with different grip widths or with the bench adjusted to different angles, thus making many different exercises possible. Machines offer a finite number of exercises, thus potentially compromising overall development.

(6) Safety

Machines are generally safer than free weights, particularly when training without a partner or spotter. Dumbbells and barbells can be dropped or plates become unsecured: machines usually allow the weight stack to be returned if you fail to complete a full repetition. When training with free weights to the point of failure, it is essential to have a spotter.

Machines are generally safer for beginners while they are developing the basic motor skills and body awareness needed to control a movement. Once they have acquired this confidence, they can include more free-weight exercises in their routine.

(7) Aesthetic appeal

Some beginners, especially women, find free weights intimidating. Machines generally have a greater aesthetic appeal and may encourage beginners to commence training. Free weights have a more macho image which may appeal to some trainers. They can encourage greater competitiveness and motivation and therefore increase strength and mass gains.

Beginning your programme

The main aim of your first few workouts is to familiarise yourself with the exercises and develop a good technique. The amount of weight you use is not important: it is best to use very light weights so you can focus on the full range of movement of each exercise. To start with, do not concentrate too much on the number of repetitions you complete, but pay attention to the quality of each set.

You should always seek the advice of a qualified instructor to show you how to perform the exercises and help you design your personal programme. If you have not used weights before or if you have not trained for a while, do not rely on written instructions – use them in conjunction with practical instruction.

Follow the basic techniques in the order described below. These will produce great results for both beginners and more experienced trainers.

Basic training methods

Circuit weight training

This method is ideal for improving overall muscle tone and strength and for familiarising yourself with the exercises. It is also good for those simply wishing to maintain muscle strength, endurance and general fitness without significantly increasing muscle mass.

Circuit training with weights comprises a series of exercises which are performed consecutively, taking relatively little rest in between. In the basic circuit, the sequence is arranged so that different muscle groups are worked in adjacent exercises. For example, leg exercises are alternated with upper body exercises. This allows you to keep going for longer before reaching fatigue on a particular muscle group, thus emphasising stamina and muscle endurance more than strength.

To increase strength, you can change the order of the exercises so that those working the same muscle groups are performed consecutively. To increase muscle endurance, you can increase the number of repetitions performed on each exercise. To increase stamina, you can increase your total workout time (e.g. the number of times you perform the circuit or the number of different exercises in each circuit) or reduce the time interval between exercises.

How often?
The American College of Sports Medicine recommend training two or three times a week on non-consecutive days. Aim to complete your workout in 30—45 minutes (excluding warm-up time). If it takes you less time, either increase the rest period between sets, add more exercises per circuit or increase the number of circuits you perform. If it takes you longer than 45 minutes, decrease any one of these factors.

How many repetitions?
Beginners should start with 10—15 reps. After four weeks, experienced trainers can change this according to their particular objectives:

(a) increasing muscle strength

Reps = 8—12

Select a weight that will allow you to complete the chosen number of reps just before your muscles reach the point of failure. The last couple should feel very difficult. Take 30—45 seconds rest between each exercise.

(b) increasing muscle endurance

Reps = 12—20

Select a weight that will allow you to complete the chosen number of reps. The last couple should feel relatively hard. Take 20—30 seconds rest between each exercise.

(c) increasing overall stamina

Reps = 15—25

Select a weight that will allow you to complete the chosen number of reps with relative ease. You should feel fairly breathless but your muscles should not 'burn' or reach the point of failure. Take 10—20 seconds rest between each exercise.

Sample circuit weight training programme

Squat	15 reps
Bench press	15 reps
Leg extension	15 reps
Shoulder press (dumbbells)	15 reps
The crunch	15 reps
Lat pulldown	15 reps
Lying leg curl	15 reps
Biceps curl	15 reps
Oblique curl up	15 reps
Triceps pushdown	15 reps
Leg press	15 reps
Upright row	15 reps
Repeat circuit 2—3 times	

Set training

This training method is a progression from circuit weight training. The number of sets of each exercise is increased from 1 to 2—6, depending on experience. Thus the training intensity is increased and a greater overload is reached, which, in turn, will produce greater increases in muscle strength and mass.

For example, to perform 3 consecutive sets of squats, select a weight that will enable you to complete 8—12 reps before reaching muscular fatigue, i.e. the point at which you can no longer lift the weight in the proper form. The last couple of reps should feel very difficult. Rest between sets until your breathing rate almost returns to normal. For the following set you can either keep the weight the same or, if necessary, reduce the weight to enable you to complete 8—12 reps.

Once you are able to perform more than 3 sets for a muscle group, you should use the split training technique (*see* page 44), training selected muscle groups in each workout. If you train your whole body using more than 3 sets for each muscle group, your total workout time will be too long and you will reach fatigue before you have completed the workout.

Example of set training (whole body)

Squat	10—15 reps	3 sets
Bench press	10—15 reps	3 sets
Shoulder press	10—15 reps	3 sets
Lat pulldown	10—15 reps	3 sets
Biceps curl	10—15 reps	3 sets
Triceps extension	10—15 reps	3 sets
The crunch	10—15 reps	3 sets

Pyramid training

During pyramid training, the weight is increased in each set and the repetitions reduced. With this method, the muscles reach greater overload. Select a weight that will enable you to reach near or complete failure at the end of each set. Take approximately 45 seconds—2 minutes rest between sets, depending on the type of exercise and the amount of weight used – enough time to allow your breathing rate to almost return to normal. Squats, for example, involve a greater energy output than, say, flyes or biceps curls so you will need to rest longer between sets.

Example of pyramid training for squats

Set 1	15 reps	40 kg
Set 2	12 reps	60 kg
Set 3	8 reps	80 kg
Set 4	6 reps	100 kg

Advanced training methods

Split training

This method increases the volume and intensity of your training. Once you have reached more than 20—25 sets overall per workout during set training, you need to begin split training, i.e. split your body parts into two or three groups and exercise only part of your body during each workout.

This will increase your training frequency from two or three to four (or more) sessions per week. However, a split routine will promote better recovery between workouts since each body part is trained less frequently. It will also produce faster hypertrophy since the volume of training for each muscle is increased.

The most fundamental split is a two-way split. This involves dividing the muscle groups in your body into two groups and exercising each group twice a week – a total of four sessions. For example, you could train chest, back and biceps on Monday and Thursday; legs, shoulders, triceps and abdominals on Tuesday and Friday. There is no hard and fast rule but, generally, you should train two major body parts and one or two smaller body parts per workout.

To increase the intensity further you can divide your body parts into three and then four groups. This method should only be used by experienced trainers, after at least 12 months of training, as it places greater demands on your recovery ability. The advantage is that it allows you to train each body part more intensely, using heavier weights or more sets, thus increasing the overload.

However, the benefits of training more frequently soon diminish once you exceed five days per week. Research suggests that less

Sample two-way split training programme

Monday and Thursday		Tuesday and Friday	
Bench press	3 sets	Squat	3 sets
Flye	3 sets	Lunge	3 sets
Incline press	3 sets	Leg curl	3 sets
Chin	3 sets	Barbell shoulder press	3 sets
Seated row	3 sets	Dumbbell lateral raise	3 sets
Close grip pulldown	3 sets	Upright row	3 sets
Biceps curl	4 sets	Triceps extension	4 sets
		The crunch	4 sets

frequent workouts (3—5 times a week) performed at high intensity (reaching overload) produce the greatest strength and mass gains. If you attempt to work out more than five days a week and/or train twice a day, a method once popularised by competitive body-builders in the 1980s, you will be at risk of overtraining, i.e. slower gains or none at all, poor recovery, susceptibility to infection and injury and chronic fatigue.

Sample four-way split training programme

Monday	Tuesday	Thursday	Friday
Bench press 3 x 8—12	Chin 3 x 8—12	Squat 3 x 8—15	Shoulder press 3 x 8—12
Incline press 3 x 8—12	Seated row 3 x 8—12	Lunge 3 x 10—15	Lateral raise 3 x 8—12
Flye 3 x 8—12	Lat pulldown behind neck 3 x 8—12	Leg extension 3 x 8—12	Upright row 3 x 8—12
Biceps curl 3 x 8—12	The crunch 2 x 20	Leg curl 4 x 8—12	Triceps extension 3 x 8—12
Preacher curl 3 x 8—12	Oblique crunch 2 x 20	Calf raise 6 x 12—15	Triceps pushdown 3 x 8—12

Eccentric training

There are two parts to an exercise: the concentric phase during which the muscle contracts or shortens; and the eccentric phase during which the muscle lengthens. For example, when performing a bench press, as you press the weight up away from your chest, the pectorals contract. This is the concentric (positive) phase of the movement. When you lower the weight back to your chest, the pectorals lengthen – the eccentric (negative) phase of the movement.

Altering your training tempo can bring about startling improvements in your training gains. The key to optimal strength development is the speed at which you complete each portion of the movement, in particular the eccentric phase. Many trainers make the mistake of lowering the weight too fast, neglecting the eccentric part of the movement. You can greatly increase your strength and mass gains by modifying your training to incorporate eccentric training.

What are the benefits of eccentric training?
Eccentric training is responsible for the greatest increases in muscle fibre growth. Many studies have demonstrated that it is the lowering phase of a movement, not the lifting, which causes maximum muscle growth (hypertrophy).

During an eccentric contraction there is more mechanical load per motor unit. As a result, eccentric training can generate significantly more tension (1.3 times greater) than concentric training. Increased tension provides a greater stimulus to the muscle fibres which, in turn, means greater strength and growth.

Eccentric training causes considerable sub-cellular muscle fibre damage: it literally tears portions of the muscle fibres. This has been shown to be responsible for the release of two prominent growth factors that stimulate muscle cells to re-build. Concentric-only training, on the other hand, does not bring about significant muscle hypertrophy or damage, although it does increase the strength of a muscle.

Is concentric training unimportant?
This is not to say that you should perform eccentric-only training or that concentric movements are a waste of time. Both eccentric and concentric movements are essential for stimulating muscle growth. Research has shown that a combined concentric-eccentric exercise leads to greater tissue damage and hence greater hypertrophy than

eccentric-only training. The concentric phase stimulates or primes the muscle for the eccentric phase. When the muscle runs out of energy during the concentric phase (i.e. you reach the point of 'failure') it locks up and you cannot move the weight any further. When you then return the weight to the starting position – the eccentric phase – the muscle fibres tear slightly, stimulating muscle growth.

How can I put eccentric training into practice?

After completing the concentric phase of an exercise, lower the weight slowly and under control, counting at least four seconds. Do not allow gravity to return it or haphazardly allow the weight to return to the weight stack. Try to resist the movement as much as possible; in fact the eccentric phase should take longer to complete than the concentric phase. The key to eccentric training is to contract or tense your muscles as you lengthen them.

So, for example, when you are performing a bench press, push the weight up until your arms are straight, pause for a moment then slowly return it to your chest counting slowly to four, and at the same time trying to resist the downward motion.

Maximum muscle fibre damage and therefore hypertrophy occurs during eccentric training following failure during the concentric phase. So, in practice, what this means is that you should complete as many reps as possible through the full range of movement, controlling the weight on the way down, then once you near failure lower the weight very slowly. With free weights, make sure you have a spotter to help you in case you lose control of the weight. You can recognise this point of near-failure: it is when most people would rack the weight and end the set. However, don't bounce the weight or lose form – get your spotter to assist during the last couple of concentric contractions if necessary, then focus on lowering the weight very slowly during the eccentric phase. This is the best time to stimulate maximum muscle growth.

How many reps and how much weight?

Since it is the fast twitch fibres which are mainly responsible for muscle growth, you need to select a weight and repetition range that ensures maximum stimulation of these fibres. This occurs in the 6—12 repetitions range. In other words, choose a weight heavy enough to cause concentric failure in this rep range. If you can complete more than 12 reps, increase the weight. If you cannot complete 6 reps fully then you need to reduce the weight.

Warm up with one or two light sets of 12—20 reps then increase the weight for a further 2—3 sets of 6—8 reps using the eccentric training technique.

How long should I allow for recovery?

Following hard eccentric training, muscle fibre damage continues for around 48 hours, before the fibres start to repair and re-build. This may take approximately 7 days to complete, so you should leave sufficient recovery time before training the same muscles. For most experienced trainers it is likely to be 5—7 days, but the exact time will depend on your workout intensity and duration and your own individual training experience. If your muscles still feel sore, this indicates that they are still damaged or healing, so you should avoid hard training until the soreness disappears. If you train the muscle before it has fully recovered, you will not be able to train as hard and thus your training gains (muscle growth and strength) will be less.

Precautions for eccentric training

◆ Enlist the help of a training partner or spotter as eccentric training can be dangerous for certain exercises.

◆ Do not 'cheat' the weight up during the concentric phase as you approach failure: you may pull or strain another muscle or damage your lower back if you use your body momentum to complete the movement, e.g. swinging backwards during biceps curls; arching your back during a bench press.

◆ Do not use eccentric training all the time. It is very intense so you should intersperse your workouts with regular training and also cycle your training methods, using eccentric training for no more than 4—6 weeks at a time.

◆ Eccentric training is not suitable for beginners as it is very intense and may lead to injury if performed incorrectly.

◆ Ensure you allow adequate recovery periods between workouts and avoid overtraining.

High rep/low rep training

To encourage maximum muscle development, you need to stress both the fast and slow twitch muscle fibres. Fast twitch fibres are used in explosive, powerful movements and fatigue quickly, after just a few seconds of all-out effort. They hypertrophy more readily than slow twitch fibres and so are largely responsible for increases in muscle mass. Thus, they are best stimulated by heavy sets and low reps (4—8).

Slow twitch fibres are involved in lower intensity, longer duration muscle contractions and can continue working for much greater periods of time, up to a few hours in some instances. They are stimulated by performing high reps (12—20).

To stimulate both fibre types therefore, you need to include high and low rep sets in your workout. For example, if you are performing lat pulldowns, complete the first two sets with a relatively light weight that allows you to do 12—20 reps. This will stimulate the slow twitch fibres. Then progressively increase the weight so that you can complete 4—8 reps before reaching failure. These sets will stimulate the fast twitch fibres.

Forced rep training

Each exercise has a 'sticking point' during the concentric phase, that is the part of the movement where gravity and unfavourable leverage make it hardest. It is usually this part of the movement at which the point of muscular failure is reached. However, you can overcome this part of the movement and complete the repetition with the assistance of a training partner, who will help you to force out another rep by applying just enough extra force to keep the weight moving through the sticking point.

You should only use this training technique for the last 1 or 2 reps of your heaviest sets. You should be able to complete at least 6 reps on your own in the correct form – if you cannot complete 6 reps, reduce the weight.

The advantage of forced rep training is that you can work past the point of muscular failure and thus increase the overload. For example, if you can normally complete 6 reps at 70 kg on the bench press, the forced rep training method enables you to complete 8 reps, thus increasing the amount of stress that your pectorals receive. This will increase hypertrophy, muscle strength and mass. Thus on your next workout you may be able to complete 7 reps on your own. Continuing to employ the forced rep training method will lead to increased improvements in strength, so that after a few weeks you may be able to lift, say, 80 kg for 6 reps.

Descending set training

This method is designed to work your muscles beyond the point of failure, thus increasing the overload. It is particularly useful if you are training without a training partner and cannot use forced rep training. It is also a good method to use during the last 1—2 sets of an exercise to provide maximum stimulation to the muscle when it is fatigued. When you reach the point of muscular failure, return the weight to its position and then reduce it. Immediately continue the set until you reach the point of failure again. You can repeat this once more if necessary.

This method is safest for exercises with dumbbells and machines since you need to be able to return the weight safely and quickly when your muscles have reached failure. Examples of suitable exercises include leg extensions, leg curls, dumbbell presses, flyes, lateral raises, dumbbell biceps curls, lat pulldowns, seated rows and triceps pushdowns.

For example, if you are performing a set of lateral raises with 10 kg dumbbells, complete as many reps as you can in strict form, say, 8. Return the dumbbells to the floor, pick up a pair of 7.5 kg dumbbells and perform as many as you can until you reach failure, say, 5. Repeat with 5 kg dumbbells.

Since this method is very fatiguing, it should only be used for selected exercises and only for the last 1—2 sets.

Superset training

Supersets include 2 or more sets of different exercises performed consecutively with no rest period between, and taken to the point of muscular failure. There are two methods of superset training:

(1) supersets for the same muscle group
(2) supersets for opposing muscle groups.

The first method involves two exercises for the same body part, for example, incline dumbbell press followed by flyes, the advantage being that the same muscle can be worked from slightly different angles, thus involving more muscle fibres and increasing the total amount of work performed. It also increases the blood flow to the muscle due to the increased energy demand, providing greater stimulation for hypertrophy. It is also good for adding variety to your routine but should not be used for every body part or workout as it is very intense and may lead to overtraining.

The second method involves performing two exercises for opposing muscle groups, for example biceps curls followed by triceps extensions, or leg extensions followed by leg curls. The advantage of this method is that the blood is kept within the same area of the body, thus encouraging a greater flow and bringing more fuel, oxygen and nutrients to the muscle. Since the rest period is eliminated, it is also a good way of reducing your workout time, particularly useful if you have only a limited time to train.

Unlike the first method, this method does not significantly increase the muscle overload. However, it does increase the demands on your cardiovascular system since the rest periods are greatly reduced, and can therefore help to improve lactic acid tolerance, raise the anaerobic threshold and develop better stamina.

Pre-exhaust training

Pre-exhaust training enables you to work the target muscle maximally. When you perform a compound exercise (e.g. bench press) the movement involves not only the prime mover, in this case the pectorals, but also a number of other smaller muscle groups, such as the triceps. The smaller muscle groups often fatigue before the prime mover reaches fatigue, limiting the amount of stimulation received by the prime mover.

With pre-exhaust training, the prime movers are partially exhausted by performing an isolation exercise prior to performing the compound exercise. For example, performing flyes before bench press works the pectorals but not the triceps so that they will fatigue before, or at the same time as, the triceps.

Training cycles

Training cycles or periodisation is an application of the principles of progressive resistance training. It is a method used to make continual improvements in performance throughout the year and thus avoid reaching plateaux. If you follow the same workout for any length of time, the body soon adapts to the constant load and your gains diminish. However, by structuring your long-term training goals in a number of training cycles, you will be able to make gains in strength, mass and definition all year round, and will avoid overtraining and injuries.

Most advanced trainers use four training cycles per year. Each cycle spans about 10 weeks and involves a gradual increase in training intensity until you reach a peak in your performance. This is usually gauged by the amount of weight that can be lifted. For example, at the beginning of your cycle the maximum weight that you can lift through one complete rep on the bench press may be 65 kg. Each week you add more weight to each set and perform fewer reps, thus increasing your training intensity and the overload, so that 10 weeks later your maximum weight has increased to, say 70 kg. Once you have attained your new 10-week maximum you can take a short rest of 1—2 weeks during which you do only very light training, or a completely different activity, before beginning the next training cycle. You then reduce your training intensity and gradually build up to your next peak.

Ideally, you can use different training cycles to develop different aspects of fitness. For example, one training cycle can be designed to develop strength and mass using basic power exercises, low reps (6—10) and heavy weights, while a second can be designed to improve muscular endurance using high reps (10—20) and lighter weights.

Yearly training cycle plan for strength (e.g. bench press)

Week	Cycle 1		Cycle 2		Cycle 3		Cycle 4	
1	50 kg	10 reps	55 kg	10 reps	60 kg	10 reps	65 kg	10 reps
2	52.5 kg	9 reps	57.5 kg	9 reps	62.5 kg	9 reps	67.5 kg	9 reps
3	55 kg	8 reps	60 kg	8 reps	65 kg	8 reps	70 kg	8 reps
4	57.5 kg	7 reps	62.5 kg	7 reps	67.5 kg	7 reps	72.5 kg	7 reps
5	60 kg	6 reps	65 kg	6 reps	70 kg	6 reps	75 kg	6 reps
6	62.5 kg	5 reps	67.5 kg	5 reps	72.5 kg	5 reps	87.5 kg	5 reps
7	65 kg	4 reps	70 kg	4 reps	75 kg	4 reps	90 kg	4 reps
8	67.5 kg	3 reps	72.5 kg	3 reps	77.5 kg	3 reps	92.5 kg	3 reps
9	70 kg	2 reps	75 kg	2 reps	80 kg	2 reps	95 kg	2 reps
10	72.5 kg	1 rep	77.5 kg	1 rep	82.5 kg	1 rep	97.5 kg	1 rep

Yearly training cycle plan for strength, mass, endurance and definition

Week	Cycle 1 Strength & mass	Cycle 2 Endurance & definition	Cycle 3 Strength & mass	Cycle 4 Endurance & definition
1	Basic exercises: e.g. squats, bench press, shoulder press, chins, dead lifts	Greater variety of isolation exercises: e.g. lunges, lateral raises, triceps kickbacks, concentration curls	Basic exercises: e.g. squats, bench press, shoulder press, chins, dead lifts	Greater variety of isolation exercises: e.g. lunges, lateral raises, triceps kickbacks, concentration curls
2				
3				
4	6—10 sets per body part		6—10 sets per body part	
5	Heavy weights	up to 12 sets per body part	Heavy weights	up to 12 sets per body part
6	6—10 reps per set	Moderate— light weights	6—10 reps per set	Moderate— light weights
7	4-way split	12—20 reps per set	4-way split	12—20 reps per set
8	Up to 2 mins rest between sets	2-way split	Up to 2 mins rest between sets	2-way split
9		20—60 secs rest between sets		20—60 secs rest between sets
10				

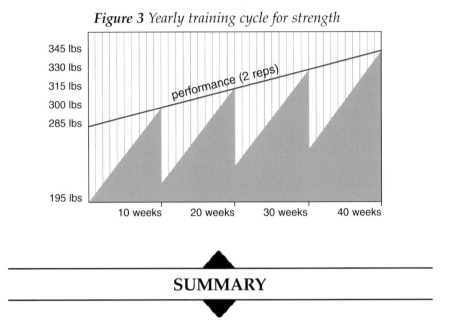

Figure 3 *Yearly training cycle for strength*

▲

SUMMARY

▼

- ◆ Muscle mass and strength increase when subjected to a progressively increasing overload. Overload can be achieved using a variety of training techniques.
- ◆ Adequate rest and recovery are a key part of any training method; insufficient rest periods between workouts will result in slow gains or none at all.
- ◆ In general, free weights offer more advantages than machines. These include improved balance, co-ordination and motor skills, favourable biomechanics and accommodation of the natural leverage of the body.
- ◆ Basic training methods include circuit weight training (suitable for beginners or for maintaining general fitness), set training and pyramid training.
- ◆ Advanced training methods, suitable for those with more than 12 months' experience, include eccentric training, high rep-low rep training, forced rep training, descending sets, supersets and pre-exhaust training. These methods help achieve greater stimulation of the muscle fibres and increase training gains.
- ◆ The use of training cycles can help make continual improvements in strength, mass and definition and avoid reaching a training plateau. Most cycles span 10 weeks and are interspersed with short periods of rest.

Body fat

Most people participating in a strength training programme are concerned with improving their appearance through increasing muscle mass and definition. The latter is achieved by reducing body fat so the shape of the muscles becomes more apparent. A low body fat percentage is, therefore, a major goal for weight trainers, bodybuilders and most competitive sportspeople.

However, low body fat levels should not be achieved at the expense of your health or your performance. This chapter looks at what is considered to be a healthy body fat level and why this varies from one individual to another. It also explains how aerobic training can help you improve your body composition and reach your required strength and muscle mass.

Body fat and physical performance

In general terms, sports performance improves as body fat reduces, and diminishes as fat accumulates, although this is not a straightforward, linear relationship. Each individual has his or her own optimal fat level at which they will perform at their best. It is therefore impossible to prescribe an ideal body fat percentage for any particular sport.

You should not aim to reduce your body fat too extensively or too quickly, however. Rapid weight loss results in diminished strength, power, muscular endurance and aerobic capacity. A drop of up to 5% in strength has been measured in athletes who have lost just 2—3% of body weight through dehydration, while a strength loss of 10% has occurred in those who lost weight through strict dieting.

Essential body fat

A certain amount of body fat is needed for peak health and performance.

The minimum amount of fat necessary to keep you alive is called *essential fat* and includes the fat which forms part of your cell membranes, brain tissue, nerve sheaths, bone marrow and the fat surrounding your internal organs, where it provides insulation, protection and cushioning against physical damage. In a healthy person, essential fat accounts for about 3% of body weight.

Sex specific fat

Women have an additional minimal fat requirement called *sex specific fat*, stored mostly in the breast area and around the hips. This fat accounts for a further 5—9% of a woman's body weight and is involved in oestrogen production, ensuring normal hormonal balance and menstrual function. Below a critical threshold of 15—20% body fat, hormonal imbalance and menstrual irregularities result, although this can be reversed once body fat levels increase.

There is also recent evidence to suggest that a certain amount of body fat in men is necessary for normal hormone production. When body fat levels drop below about 5%, testosterone production decreases and the sperm count is reduced.

Storage fat

Fat is an important energy store, providing 9 kcal/g. It is used during aerobic activities such as sleeping, sitting, standing and walking, as well as during most types of exercise. This fat comes from adipose tissue distributed all over the body and also from the fat within muscle cells (this is particularly important during exercise).

It is impossible to selectively spot reduce fat from adipose tissue sites. The body uses fat from all sites, although the exact pattern of fat utilisation and storage is determined by your genetic make-up and hormonal balance.

What is a healthy level of body fat?

For peak health, doctors and physiologists recommend a minimum of 5% body fat for men and 10% for women; however a generally healthy range is between 13% and 18% for men and between 18%

and 25% for women. Most élite sportspeople have a lower body fat than this recommended range, typically between 4—10% in men and 13—18% in women, the lowest levels being found in competitive bodybuilders who often maintain the minimum level needed for survival! While such low body fat percentages may be desirable for improving athletic performance and aesthetics, they are not necessarily compatible with peak health.

The problems with body fat levels of below 15—20% in women include the development of hormonal imbalances, reduced oestrogen production, irregular menstruation (*oligomenorrhoea*), menstrual dysfunction, the cessation of periods (*amenorrhoea*) and infertility. Therefore, a woman's chances of becoming pregnant are drastically reduced if she has a very low body fat level. Low oestrogen levels also lead to bone mineral loss, osteopoenia, which is similar to osteoporosis. Osteoporosis usually affects post-menopausal women, however low oestrogen levels also increase the risk of it developing at an earlier age.

For men, low body fat levels (below 5%) have been shown to reduce testosterone production, sperm count, libido and sexual activity!

These hormonal changes are usually reversible when body fat levels are restored to a healthy range; however, the long-term effects on bone health and future fertility are unknown.

Body fat and genetics

Researchers believe that we all have our own body fat 'set point', a range of body fat at which our bodies happily settle. This is genetically determined and cannot easily be changed. In addition, scientists have discovered a gene sequence (the so-called *obesity gene*) that controls body fat levels via appetite and metabolic rate. Those with a defective gene have an impaired appetite control mechanism and are more likely to overeat and put on weight.

Research suggests that body fat levels are controlled by a kind of thermostat (adipostat) in the brain which is set to a particular fat level. If your body fat level rises above your genetically set range, the fat cells produce more leptin, a chemical messenger. This signals to the brain that body fat levels are too high, so the adipostat responds by increasing the metabolic rate and reducing the appetite. Similarly, if your body fat level drops below the set range, leptin production is reduced, your metabolic rate slows down and your appetite increases in an attempt to stabilise your body fat around the set point.

This is why weight loss often slows down or 'plateaus' after a certain period of dieting – your body is attempting to keep your body fat within the genetic set range. This set range is different for every individual which may explain why some people are able to achieve a low body fat more easily than others.

◆ *Leptin and fat loss* ◆

Leptin is a protein produced by the fat cells. It plays a key role in monitoring and controlling body fat and energy balance. Scientists believe that a defective obesity gene causes the feedback mechanism described above to go awry, making the body think that it is still hungry because the signal has been interrupted.

Researchers at Rockerfeller University in New York and the Howard Hughes Medical Institute found that obese mice injected with human leptin lost weight, and it is possible that leptin may be developed as an obesity drug in the future. It would only be appropriate for use with obese people, however, not for those less than 30 lbs overweight.

Therefore, if you attempt to reduce your body fat to an unrealistic level, you could be fighting your genes. Your appetite will increase and your metabolic rate will decrease, making it even harder to achieve your goal.

To avoid this problem, it is important to set yourself a realistic body fat goal that is compatible with your genetic fat range. If you find yourself continually reaching a sticking point when dieting, this is probably the lower end of your fat range and you should not go below this. To do so would involve prolonged dieting which could put your health at risk.

Low body fat and undernutrition

To reduce your body fat below the set range you would have to continue reducing your calorie intake further and further. This inevitably means a reduced intake of carbohydrate, vitamins and minerals.

A low carbohydrate diet quickly results in depleted glycogen stores which, in turn, lead to poor energy levels, reduced capacity for exercise, fatigue, poor recovery between workouts and eventual burn-out. A low carbohydrate intake also increases protein break-down – causing loss of muscle mass and strength – just the opposite of what you are aiming for through your fitness programme. Loss of muscle mass, or failure to increase muscle mass, despite hard training, is very common when trainers attempt to achieve very low body fat levels. Once body fat levels and glycogen stores get too low, lean tissue is broken down to supply the necessary energy. The result – muscle loss!

Prolonged dieting and very low fat intake can lead to other nutritional problems. Your intake of the essential fatty acids (linoleic acid and linolenic acid) will be reduced and may, in the long term, lead to essential fatty acid deficiency – dull flaky skin and other skin problems, cold extremities, reduced prostaglandin (hormone) levels leading to reduced immune function, poor control of blood pressure, vasoconstriction, blood clotting and increased PMS symptoms in women. These fatty acids are found in vegetable oils, seeds, nuts and oily fish; include at least one portion of any of these in your daily diet to avoid deficiency (*see* page 208).

Vitamin and mineral intake is generally proportional to total calorie and food intake, so as you reduce your calories your vitamin and mineral intake decreases. Fat-soluble vitamins A, D and E are found only in foods containing fat or oil so a fat-free diet will substantially reduce your intake of these vitamins. More importantly, fat is required for their absorption so taking a supplement is not the answer.

How much fat should I eat?

The International Conference on Foods, Nutrition and Sports Performance recommended a fat intake of between 15% and 30% of calories for sportspeople. This is in line with the maximum recommended by the World Health Organisation (30% of calories) and the UK government (33—35% of calories).

Your daily diet should therefore contain a minimum of 15% calories from fats and oils. For example, if you consume 2000 calories you should eat 33—66 g fat a day; if you eat 3000 calories you should eat 50—100 g. Your fat intake should come mainly from unsaturated fats found in vegetable oils (e.g. olive oil, rapeseed oil, sunflower oil) and products made with them (e.g. salad dressing, margarine, stir fry dishes), oily fish (e.g. sardines, mackerel, salmon), nuts, peanut and other nut butters, and avocado.

Aerobic training for weight trainers

It was once believed that aerobic training was counterproductive to a weight training programme, burning muscle and preventing gains in muscle mass. This myth has been firmly disproved; in fact, aerobic training provides numerous benefits for weight trainers, as described below:

- ◆ reduces body fat/maintains low body fat percentage
- ◆ increases the body's fat burning capacity during exercise and rest
- ◆ improves body composition
- ◆ increases cardiovascular fitness (stamina)
- ◆ reduces stress and anxiety
- ◆ improves confidence, self esteem and mood
- ◆ reduces blood pressure, blood cholesterol and risk of heart disease.

What is the difference between aerobic and anaerobic exercise?

'Aerobic' literally means 'with oxygen'. Most everyday activities such as sleeping, sitting and walking are aerobic in nature, as oxygen is being used to provide energy. Aerobic exercise such as jogging, stepping, cycling or swimming, increases the body's demand for oxygen. Aerobic exercise can be maintained for a relatively long period of time and is performed at a relatively low level of intensity (less than 85% of maximal heart rate – *see* page 62). Aerobic activities are fuelled mainly by glycogen, glucose and fat – the lower the intensity and the longer the exercise continues the greater the proportion of fat used in the fuel mixture. Aerobically-trained people are also able to use more fat than untrained people at any given intensity.

Anaerobic exercise uses energy produced without oxygen. This comes from either phosphocreatine (the body's high-energy compound that generates ATP very rapidly), or a mixture of phosphocreatine, glucose and glycogen, depending on the exercise intensity. Activities involving short bursts of high-intensity explosive exercise such as sprinting, jumping, kicking, hitting, throwing and heavy weight training/lifting which can only be kept up for a few seconds are fuelled by the phosphocreatine energy system. Activities lasting 30—90 seconds, such as heavy weight training or 400-metre sprinting are fuelled by phosphocreatine, blood glucose and muscle glycogen. Fats cannot be broken down in the absence of oxygen and are, therefore, not used for anaerobic exercise.

How does aerobic training reduce your fat stores?

Regular aerobic exercise enhances the body's ability to burn fat for energy both at rest and during activity. Not only do you burn extra fat calories during aerobic exercise but regular training increases the number of enzymes involved in fat metabolism, a natural adaptation that has a long-term effect on your body's metabolism.

For example, there is an increase in the enzymes which break down fat (stored as triglycerides in adipose tissue) into its component fatty acids. These fatty acids are released into the bloodstream and transported as lipoproteins to other tissues such as muscle where they are needed for energy production. The fatty acids are then taken up by the muscle cells, transferred into the mitochondria and broken down into ATP. Thus, aerobic training increases enzyme production and the body's ability to break down fat.

The more aerobically fit you are, the greater the percentage of fat you can break down at any exercise intensity. Just as you can train your muscles to become stronger and bigger, so you can train your aerobic system to burn fat more efficiently. Including aerobic training in your weight training programme will therefore help you to achieve and maintain a lower body fat percentage and better muscle definition.

Aerobic exercise guidelines

How much?
The Health Education Authority recommend a minimum of 20 minutes of vigorous aerobic activity (burning at least 7.5 kcal/min) repeated three times a week in order to build up aerobic fitness. Alternatively, 30 minutes of moderate activity (burning 5—7.5 kcal/min) repeated five times a week is recommended in order to reduce the risk of heart disease and maintain a basic fitness level.

When?

This depends on your individual metabolism and lifestyle. Choose a time of day that fits in well with your daily schedule; that way you will be less likely to miss a workout. Research suggests that it may be better to split your aerobic training and weight training into separate sessions to minimise catabolism (breakdown of lean mass). If you prefer to do both in one session, complete your weight training workout first when glycogen stores are high.

Which activity?

The choice of activity depends on your personal preference, and the equipment and time available to you. For example, if your time is limited, choose a higher intensity (vigorous) activity – expending at least 7.5 kcal/min – which makes you feel as if you are working very hard and leaves you almost out of breath. If time constraints are less important and you prefer exercising at a slower, steadier rate, choose a lower intensity (moderate) activity which feels fairly hard work but does not leave you out of breath.

Aerobic activity should be rhythmic, it should involve your large muscle groups, e.g. legs, and be sustained for at least 20 minutes in your training zone (*see* below). Suitable high-intensity/vigorous aerobic activities include:

◆ running/treadmill
◆ fitness/power walking
◆ stepping machine/stair climber
◆ cycling/stationary bicycle
◆ swimming
◆ aerobic classes/aqua aerobics/step aerobics/slide aerobics
◆ climbing machine
◆ rowing/rowing machine.

How hard?

To improve your aerobic fitness, your heart rate needs to be maintained between 60—85% of your maximum heart rate (MHR). This range is called the target heart rate zone. To find your MHR, subtract your age from 220. For example, if you are aged 30:

MHR = 220 − 30 = 190

Target heart rate training zone = 60% x 190—85% x 190
$$= 114—162$$

High or low intensity?

This depends on your goals and your fitness level. Although fat provides a greater percentage of energy during low-intensity exercise, you still have to take account of the total calories burned. For example, walking for 60 minutes will burn 270 kcal, of which 60% (160 kcal) come from fat, while jogging for 60 minutes will burn 680 kcal, of which 40% (270 kcal) come from fat. Thus, the higher intensity exercise results in a greater fat loss over the same period of time.

Studies have shown that a shorter period (e.g. 40 minutes) of high-intensity exercise burns about the same amount of fat as a longer period (e.g. 60 minutes) of low-intensity exercise. So, if time is a premium, shorter periods of high-intensity exercise will give you the same results in terms of fat loss as longer periods of low-intensity exercise. On the other hand, low-intensity exercise is often more suitable for beginners who may not be fit enough to embark on a high-intensity programme. Also, low-intensity exercise is more accessible and enjoyable for many people who are therefore more likely to continue the exercise programme.

In summary, if fat loss is your main goal, choose high-intensity aerobic exercise if you are sufficiently fit and enjoy doing it, or if you have only a short time to work out. Choose longer periods of low-intensity exercise if you are less fit or find it more enjoyable than high-intensity exercise.

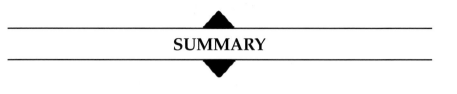

SUMMARY

- ◆ Muscle definition depends on body fat percentage, in particular subcutaneous fat, and is therefore increased by reducing total body fat.
- ◆ There is a minimum body fat requirement for health and performance consisting of essential fat (structural fat); sex specific fat (hormonal production and regulation); storage fat (energy production).
- ◆ The recommended body fat range for general health is 13—18% for men and 18—25% for women. Sportspeople and weight trainers often attain lower levels.
- ◆ In women, very low body fat levels (below 15—20%) can lead to hormonal imbalances, reduced oestrogen production, menstrual dysfunction, amenorrhoea, infertility, bone mineral loss and increased risk of osteoporosis.
- ◆ In men, very low body fat levels (below 5%) can reduce testosterone production, sperm count and libido.
- ◆ Prolonged dieting can result in low nutrient intakes (in particular essential fatty acids), depleted nutrient stores and glycogen levels, fatigue, muscle loss, and reduced performance.
- ◆ There is evidence that everyone has a genetically determined body fat range, maintained via the production of leptin and controlled by an adipostat in the brain which alters basal metabolic rate and appetite.
- ◆ Aerobic exercise will help achieve and maintain low body fat levels, improve muscle definition and body composition, and provide numerous health benefits.
- ◆ Shorter periods of high-intensity aerobic exercise are equally or more effective than longer periods of low-intensity aerobic exercise in reducing body fat.

Muscle fuel

Carbohydrate, in the form of blood glucose and muscle glycogen, is the main fuel used during strength training, and it is therefore crucial that you optimise your carbohydrate stores prior to every workout.

Training with low blood glucose and glycogen stores means that you will suffer fatigue quicker and find it harder to continue exercising. Your workout becomes less intense, reducing the training stimulus and gains. Over consecutive workouts, this can lead to symptoms of overtraining – chronic fatigue and decreased immune system.

Calculating your carbohydrate requirement

The International Conference on Foods, Nutrition & Performance (1991) recommended a diet containing 60—70% energy from carbohydrate. Work out your carbohydrate intake in one of two ways.

(1) From your calorie intake
Estimate your calorie (energy) intake over a minimum of three days using food/calorie tables. Multiply this figure by 60% and divide by 4 to give you your recommended carbohydrate intake in grams.

For example: energy intake = 2500 calories
energy from carbohydrate = 2500 x 60% = 1500
g carbohydrate = 1500 / 4 = 375 g

(2) From your body weight and activity
Calculate your daily carbohydrate requirement using the chart overleaf which is based on body weight and activity level, then multiply this by your weight in kilogrammes.

For example, if you weigh 85 kg and are moderately active (1 hour of exercise per day):

carbohydrate requirement = 85 x 6 = 510 g/day

Daily carbohydrate requirement

Activity level*	g carbohydrate/kg/day
Light (< 1h/day)	4—5
Light—moderate (approx. 1h/day)	5—6
Moderate (1—2h/day)	6—7
Moderate—heavy (2—4h/day)	7—8
Heavy (> 4h/day)	8—10
*Number of hours of medium-intensity exercise or sport	

Use the box below to help you plan your meals and snacks and achieve your recommended carbohydrate intake. For example, 10 portions of foods would give you approximately 500 g carbohydrate.

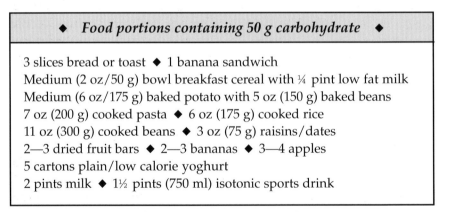

◆ **Food portions containing 50 g carbohydrate** ◆

3 slices bread or toast ◆ 1 banana sandwich
Medium (2 oz/50 g) bowl breakfast cereal with ¼ pint low fat milk
Medium (6 oz/175 g) baked potato with 5 oz (150 g) baked beans
7 oz (200 g) cooked pasta ◆ 6 oz (175 g) cooked rice
11 oz (300 g) cooked beans ◆ 3 oz (75 g) raisins/dates
2—3 dried fruit bars ◆ 2—3 bananas ◆ 3—4 apples
5 cartons plain/low calorie yoghurt
2 pints milk ◆ 1½ pints (750 ml) isotonic sports drink

Re-fuelling

You should start re-fuelling as soon as possible after exercise, as glycogen production and storage is faster during the two hours immediately following a workout, increasing from the normal 5% to 7—8% per hour. Therefore, eating carbohydrate during this period allows you to re-fuel and recover faster prior to your next workout.

Aim to eat at least 1 g carbohydrate/kg body weight in this post-exercise period. For example, if you weigh 80 kg, aim to eat a minimum of 80 g carbohydrate (e.g. ½ pint isotonic drink and one banana sandwich). For efficient glycogen re-fuelling you should continue to eat at least 50 g carbohydrate every two hours either in solid or liquid form, so meals or snacks should be planned at frequent and regular intervals. If you leave long gaps without eating, glycogen storage and recovery will be slower. Similarly, if you eat most of your carbohydrate in just one or two large meals, storage will be less efficient and some of the carbohydrate may be converted into body fat.

The length of time that it takes to re-fuel after your workout depends on three factors.

(1) The intensity and duration of the workout

The higher the intensity of your training session and the longer it takes to complete, the more glycogen you use and the more depleted your muscle glycogen stores. Depletion occurs both after a long aerobic training session (more than 90 minutes of exercise performed at 60—80% VO_2 max) and a short, highly intense training session (as little as 15—30 minutes of extremely intense weight training/multiple sprint training), so you need to allow an adequate rest period to re-fuel your muscles before training the same muscle group again.

(2) The amount and frequency of carbohydrate intake

For fast and efficient glycogen re-fuelling it is important to eat the right amount of carbohydrate and to consume it at regular intervals during the day. As your carbohydrate intake increases, so the rate of glycogen storage increases (*see* fig. 4, on page 68).

This is a particularly important factor if you train over four times a week. If you fail to eat enough carbohydrate, re-fuelling and recovery will take longer, and if you train before your glycogen stores are fully replenished, you will not be able to train as hard or for as long, you will fatigue sooner and achieve smaller training improvements.

Figure 4 *Glycogen storage depends on carbohydrate intake*

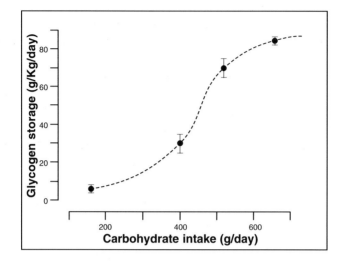

(3) Training experience

With training, your ability to store glycogen increases by up to 20%, and glycogen re-fuelling becomes more efficient. In other words, the more training experience you have in your sport and the higher your fitness level, the faster your muscles can re-fuel and the more glycogen can be stored – it would therefore take a beginner longer to replace his glycogen stores than it would an experienced trainer eating the same amount of carbohydrate.

Types of carbohydrate

Carbohydrates can be divided into two categories: *simple* (sugars) and *complex* (starches and fibre). These terms simply refer to the number of sugar units in the molecule, and both are useful for fuelling the muscles during exercise.

Simple carbohydrates include:
◆ **glucose** – found naturally in fruit and honey. All carbohydrates are broken down in the digestive system into glucose. It is the main form in which carbohydrates are transported in the blood-stream, and can be referred to as blood sugar.

- **fructose (fruit sugar)** – found in fruit and honey. It is the sweetest-tasting sugar. It is a slow-releasing sugar because it first has to be converted into glucose in the liver.
- **sucrose (ordinary packet sugar)** – made up of one unit of glucose and one unit of fructose. It is found in large quantities in sugar cane and sugar beet as well as in most fruit and vegetables.
- **lactose (milk sugar)** – found only in milk and dairy products. It is made up of one unit of glucose and one unit of galactose and is about one third as sweet as sucrose.
- **glucose or corn syrup** – produced commercially from the breakdown of cornstarch into glucose and is used in jam and bakery products such as biscuits and cakes.

Maltodextrins or glucose polymers are short chains of 3—20 glucose units. They are produced commercially from the partial breakdown of cornstarch and do not taste sweet. They are closer to a sugar than a starch in terms of their structure, and are used in sports drinks, commercial desserts, soups, and baby foods.

Complex carbohydrates include starches and non-starch polysaccharides (dietary fibre). They are made up of thousands of simple sugar units linked together.

In practice, many foods contain a mixture of both simple and complex carbohydrates. For example, biscuits and cakes contain flour (complex) and sugar (simple). Bananas contain a mixture of sugars and starches depending on their degree of ripeness.

From a physiological point of view you can fuel muscles with either simple or complex carbohydrates. All are broken down into single sugars and can equally well be converted into glycogen. The choice of carbohydrate therefore depends on the following.

(1) The nutritional value

In general, foods containing complex carbohydrates (e.g. bread and grains) and the 'naturally occurring' simple carbohydrates (e.g. fruit and milk) have a better nutritional value than foods rich in refined simple carbohydrates (e.g. soft drinks and confectionery). So, in practice, aim to get most of your carbohydrates from foods providing a good range of nutrients, i.e. bread, grains, cereals, starchy vegetables, pulses, fruit and dairy products.

Carbohydrate categories of various foods

Foods high in simple carbohydrates	Foods high in complex carbohydrates	Foods containing a mixture of simple and complex carbohydrates
Sugar (white and brown)	Flour (brown and white)	Cakes
Jam, honey and other	Bread (all types)	Biscuits
preserves	Pasta, rice and noodles	Breakfast cereals
Fruit (fresh, dried or	Oats and other grains	(sweetened)
tinned)	Breakfast cereals	Puddings
Yoghurt	(without sugar)	Sweet pastries, pies,
Fromage frais	Pulses (beans, lentils,	flans
Ice cream	peas)	Cheesecake
Jelly	Potatoes, yams, sweet	Bananas
Confectionery	potatoes, eddoes	
Milk	Plantains (green	
Soft drinks	bananas)	
	Parsnips	
	Sweetcorn	

(2) The glycaemic index

The glycaemic index (GI) is a measure of the speed of carbohydrate absorption and of the resulting rate of rise in blood sugar (*see* page 71). Sometimes it is beneficial to consume fast-releasing carbohydrates; other times slow-releasing carbohydrates are preferable.

(3) The bulk

High fibre foods are filling and add considerable bulk to the diet, a potential problem for trainers with high calorie and carbohydrate requirements. A diet high in complex and fibre-rich carbohydrates can make it difficult to eat enough food to satisfy your daily requirements. For example, if you need 3000 kcal per day you would need to eat the equivalent of 32 shredded wheat or 11 tins of baked beans to obtain the recommended intake of 450 g carbohydrate! Therefore a mixture of complex and simple carbohydrates, and high and low fibre foods may be more suitable for those with high calorie requirements.

The glycaemic index

Every food produces a change in blood sugar levels. The glycaemic index of a food is a measure of its blood-sugar-raising ability and is technically defined as the rise in blood sugar produced after eating a food containing 50 g carbohydrate, compared with a reference food (either glucose or white bread) containing 50 g carbohydrate which is assigned a value of 100. Therefore, the closer the GI of a food is to 100, the faster the rise in blood sugar produced. Most foods have a GI of between 20—100.

At certain times it is necessary to consume carbohydrates that can be quickly absorbed and transported to the muscles, for example immediately before exercise, during strenuous exercise and in the two-hour post-exercise period. At other times, it is desirable to consume carbohydrates that are absorbed more slowly. Such occasions include the 2—4 hour period before exercise and the recovery period between workouts.

There are many factors which determine the GI of a food. It is not related to whether the carbohydrate is simple or complex – contrary to popular belief, complex carbohydrates are not necessarily absorbed more slowly than simple carbohydrates; potatoes for example (mostly complex), produce a rapid blood sugar rise, while apples (simple) produce a slow blood sugar rise.

The GI of a food depends on the following:

◆ fibre – soluble fibre reduces the blood sugar rise
◆ fat – fat slows the digestion and absorption of any food and therefore reduces the blood sugar rise. For example, bread with butter results in a slower blood sugar rise than bread eaten on its own. Fat-free foods raise blood sugar and insulin levels even higher
◆ protein – reduces the blood sugar rise
◆ the type of starch – for example, starch in beans produces a slower blood sugar rise than starch in bread
◆ cooking and processing – foods which have been processed or cooked produce a faster rise in blood sugar. For example, milling and grinding grains breaks down the cell walls and reduces the size of the starch molecules, thus allowing easier access to the digestive enzymes. The faster the food is digested the faster it is absorbed into the bloodstream and the quicker blood sugar levels go up.

The box below classifies foods as having a high (60—100), medium (40—60) or low (< 40) GI compared with glucose (100). These values relate to the consumption of single foods on an empty stomach, and can be greatly modified if eaten with other foods as part of a meal. For example, bread eaten on its own has a high GI but when eaten with cheese or baked beans, the resultant GI will be lower. Therefore, use the following GI values as a rough guide only.

The glycaemic index of various foods (Glucose = 100)

High (60—100)	GI	Moderate (40—60)	GI	Low (< 40)	GI
Cereals		**Cereals**		**Pulses**	
White bread	69	Wholemeal pasta	42	Butter beans	36
Wholemeal bread	72	White pasta	50	Baked beans	40
Brown rice	80	Oats	49	Haricot beans	31
White rice	82	Barley	22	Chick peas	36
				Lentils	29
				Kidney beans	29
				Soya beans	15
Breakfast cereals		**Breakfast cereals**			
Cornflakes	80	Porridge	54		
Muesli	66	All bran	51		
Shredded wheat	67				
Weetabix	75				
Fruit		**Fruit**		**Fruit**	
Raisins	64	Grapes	44	Apples	39
Bananas	62	Oranges	40	Cherries	23
				Plums	25
				Apricots	30
				Grapefruit	26
				Peaches	29
Vegetables		**Vegetables**		**Dairy products**	
Sweetcorn	59	Sweet potatoes	48	Milk	32
Parsnips	97	Crisps	51	Yoghurt	36
Baked potato	98	Yams	51	Ice-cream	36
Carrots	92				
Other		**Other**		**Other**	
Biscuits	59	Oatmeal biscuits	54	Fructose	20
Chocolate bar	68	Sponge cake	46		
Honey	87				
Sucrose	59				
Glucose	100				
Orange cordial	66				

Carbohydrates between workouts

Between workouts, it is beneficial to consume food with a low glycaemic index, to allow efficient and continuous glycogen storage. You are not limited to carbohydrates with a low GI however; it is possible to lower the GI of a food by combining it with other foods, for example:

◆ choose carbohydrates which are not highly processed e.g. pulses, whole fruit (rather than juice), wholegrain bread made from coarse or stoneground flour, pasta or oatmeal
◆ combine carbohydrates with some protein or fat as this will slow down their absorption. For example, eat bread with a little peanut butter, cheese, or in a sandwich with tuna or chicken. Add beans, cheese or yoghurt to baked potatoes.

Pre-exercise carbohydrates

Contrary to popular belief, pre-exercise carbohydrates can help you to maintain higher blood sugar levels, delay fatigue, improve endurance and therefore train harder for longer.

It is now known that exercise does not trigger a surge of insulin which would lower blood sugar levels. During exercise, adrenaline and other hormones are produced which actually suppress insulin, allowing blood sugar levels to be maintained. This in turn helps to maintain energy output, spare muscle glycogen, and improve performance.

Consume approximately 50 g carbohydrate 5—30 minutes before exercise but at least two hours after your last meal. Experiment with different amounts of carbohydrate and different time intervals to find the strategy that suits you best.

Carbohydrates during exercise

Researchers at California State University have found that gains in muscle strength and size are greater if blood sugar levels are kept high during strength workouts. Consuming carbohydrate during your workout may also help delay fatigue and maintain your performance, particularly in the latter stages. University of Texas researchers recommend an intake of between 30—60 g carbohydrate per hour depending on your body weight and your exercise intensity.

Any carbohydrate with a high glycaemic index would be suitable at this stage but many people find liquids easier to consume than solids. Isotonic sports drinks or carbohydrate (glucose polymer) drinks are beneficial as they serve to replenish fluid and prevent dehydration as well as supplying the necessary carbohydrate.

If you prefer solid food, choose high GI foods such as energy bars, bananas, dried fruit bars, or raisins; have a drink of water, too.

Suitable pre- or post-exercise snacks supplying 50 g carbohydrate*
2—3 bananas
1½ pints (750 ml) isotonic sports drink
3 oz (75 g) dried fruit
Jam sandwich (2 slices bread with 2 tbsp jam)
5 rice cakes with 1 banana
2½ oz (65 g) breakfast cereal
1 confectionery bar
½ pint (250 ml) glucose polymer drink (20% carbohydrate)
*Accompany solid foods with a large glass of water

What carbohydrate to eat and when?

	Before exercise	During exercise	After exercise	Between workouts
How much?	50 g	30—60 g	1 g/kg body weight	60% of energy
Time period	5—30 mins	Begin after 30 mins; regular intervals	0—2 hours	Minimum 4—6 meals/snacks
GI	High	High	High	Low—moderate
Examples	2—3 bananas ½ pint (250 ml) isotonic sports drink & 1 banana 3 oz (75 g) dried fruit 2 thick slices bread	1—2 pints (500—1000ml) sports drink/ diluted squash (3—6%) Energy bar 2—3 bananas 2—3 oz (50—75 g) dried fruit	Banana sandwich 3 oz (75 g) raisins 2 slices toast and low fat yoghurt ½ pint (250 ml) glucose polymer drink (20%) 8 oz (225 g) potato	Pasta with cheese/chicken/ fish Rice with beans Noodles with tofu/poultry/ seafood Beans on toast Potato with cottage cheese/ tuna

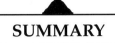

SUMMARY

- Carbohydrate is the main fuel used by muscles during strength training. It is recommended that carbohydrates provide 60—70% of energy or 5—10 g/kg body weight/day, depending on your activity level.
- Re-fuelling should begin as soon as possible after training. Glycogen manufacture increases from 5% to 7—8% per hour during the two-hour post-workout period.
- The length of time it takes to re-fuel depends on the intensity and duration of the workout, the amount and timing of carbohydrate eaten, and your training experience.
- The choice of carbohydrate depends on its nutritional package, its glycaemic index and its bulk. Whether it is complex or simple has little bearing on its ability to increase blood sugar or glycogen levels.
- The glycaemic index of a food is a measure of its blood-sugar-raising ability. It depends on the presence of other nutrients (e.g. fat, fibre and protein), the type of starch and the physical state of the food (e.g. processed or cooked).
- For efficient glycogen re-fuelling, foods with a low GI should be eaten between workouts.
- Pre-exercise carbohydrates with a high GI can help maintain blood sugar levels, delay fatigue and increase workout intensity.
- During highly intense workouts lasting for one hour or more, consuming 30—60 g high GI carbohydrate will help delay fatigue and increase performance.

8

Weight management (1): fat loss programme

Strength training and diet both play major roles in a fat loss programme. The only way to reduce body fat is to achieve a negative energy balance; that is, your energy expenditure – calories burned through basal metabolism, dietary thermogenesis and physical activity – must be greater than your energy intake – calories provided by food and drink (*see* below).

◆ ***Energy balance equations*** ◆

Energy Balance

Energy Intake	=	*Energy Expenditure*
(Food and drink)		(Basal metabolism,
		dietary thermogenesis,
		physical activity)
Result	=	*Weight maintenance*

Positive Energy Balance

Energy Intake	>	*Energy Expenditure*
(Food and drink)		(Basal metabolism,
		dietary thermogenesis,
		physical activity)
Result	=	*Weight gain*

Negative Energy Balance

Energy Intake	<	*Energy Expenditure*
(Food and drink)		(Basal metabolism,
		dietary thermogenesis,
		physical activity)
Result	=	*Weight loss*

A negative energy balance may be achieved by reducing your energy (calorie) intake, increasing your physical activity or through a combination of both of these methods. Research has shown that both endurance and strength exercise plus a reduction in energy intake produces greater fat loss and favourable changes in body composition than either endurance exercise or diet alone. It is also far more likely to produce long-term success. 95% of dieters regain their lost weight within five years so, clearly, dieting alone does not result in permanent weight loss. In fact, for most people dieting compounds rather than corrects one of the most important causes of weight gain – muscle loss, leading to a lower basal metabolic rate (BMR).

Objectives of a fat loss programme:

◆ to reduce body fat percentage
◆ to maintain muscle mass (avoid muscle loss)
◆ to maintain muscle strength
◆ to maintain energy levels
◆ to avoid a significant reduction in basal metabolic rate.

Dietary goals

Calorie intake should be reduced mainly by cutting down on fat. However, it is important to consume a small amount of fat/oil to ensure an adequate intake of essential fatty acids and fat-soluble vitamins. A minimum of 15% and a maximum of 25% calories from fat is recommended.

It is also important to maintain a high carbohydrate intake, at least 60% of calorie intake. A low carbohydrate diet may produce a rapid loss of weight initially, but this is mainly due to a decrease in your liver and muscle glycogen stores and the water that is bound to the glycogen.

Therefore, if you reduce your carbohydrate intake too much this will result in:

◆ lethargy
◆ glycogen depletion
◆ fatigue
◆ reduced training intensity and low performance
◆ increased appetite
◆ increased protein (muscle) breakdown and lean mass loss
◆ negative mental state.

Finally, a protein intake of approximately 1.4—1.7 g/kg body weight/day is necessary in order to maintain body protein and muscle mass during weight loss. However, the percentage of energy from protein increases automatically due to the reduction in fat intake.

Strength training and weight control

Strength training plays a key part in weight control for two main reasons. Firstly, it prevents the age-related reduction in metabolic rate and, secondly, it maintains or increases muscle mass.

Most people lose about ½ lb of muscle per year, which is largely responsible for the slow-down in basal metabolic rate. This is because muscle is metabolically active tissue – one pound of muscle burns 30—50 kcal a day just to maintain its mass. Strength training can prevent this muscle loss, and as more muscle means a higher metabolic rate, so more calories are used for tissue maintenance rather than being converted into fat.

In a study conducted by Wayne Westcott at the South Shore YMCA, Massachusetts, 72 overweight adults were placed into two groups. Both followed a diet comprising 60% carbohydrate, 20% fat and 20% protein. One group performed endurance exercises for 30 minutes a day, three days a week, for eight weeks; the other group performed 15 minutes of endurance exercises and 15 minutes of strength training, three days a week for eight weeks. Those performing endurance exercises only lost 3 lbs of fat and ½ lb of muscle. The endurance plus strength training group lost 10 lbs of fat and gained 2 lbs of muscle.

A further study on 25 women was based on the American College of Sports Medicine's strength training guidelines: 3 sessions a week, 1 set per exercise, 10 repetitions for 8 different exercises. After 8 weeks, their body weight remained the same but body fat was reduced by 1.9% (from 26.3% to 24.4%); they lost 2.6 lbs of fat and gained 2.7 lbs of muscle – a net improvement of 5.3 lbs in body composition.

Fat loss strategy

Set realistic goals

Before embarking on a weight loss plan, write down your goals clearly and precisely. Research has proven that writing down your intentions is far more likely to turn them into actions than thinking or talking about them.

Your goals should be S.M.A.R.T. (*see* page 12).

Monitor body composition changes

Monitoring changes in measurements at specific sites of the body allows you to see how your shape is changing and where most fat is being lost. This is more accurate than using weighing scales.

The best way to monitor your progress is by a combination of simple girth or circumference measurements (e.g. chest, waist, hips, arms, legs) and skinfold thickness measurements obtained by calipers. Exercise physiologists recommend keeping a record of skinfold thickness measurements rather than converting them into body fat percentage. This is because the conversion charts are based on equations for average, sedentary people and may not be appropriate for sportspeople or very lean or fat individuals.

Aim to lose 1—2 lbs of fat per week

Weighing yourself weekly or fortnightly can be useful for checking the speed of weight/fat loss, but do not rely exclusively on this method as it does not reflect changes in body composition. Avoid more frequent weighing as this can lead to an obsession with weight. Total weight loss may be as much as 4—5 lbs in the first week, but this is mostly in the form of glycogen and its accompanying fluid (1 lb of glycogen is stored with up to 4 lbs of water). Afterwards, aim to lose no more than 2 lbs of fat per week. If weight loss is faster, this usually suggests a loss of lean tissue so you should increase your calorie intake by 250—500 per day to slow down weight loss to a healthier level.

Keep a food diary

A food diary is a written record of your daily food and drink intake. It is a very good way to evaluate your present eating habits and find out exactly what, why, where and when you are eating. It will allow you to check whether your diet is well balanced or lacking in any important nutrients, and to take a careful look at your meal patterns and lifestyle.

Weigh and write down everything you eat and drink for at least three consecutive days – ideally for seven days. Every biscuit, spoonful of sugar in tea, scrape of butter on bread should be recorded. The period should include at least one weekend day, and it is important not to change your usual diet in any way! (*See* page 81.)

Estimate calorie, carbohydrate, fat and protein intake

You can carry out a basic dietary analysis with the help of a food composition book such as McCance & Widdowson's *Composition of Foods*, The *MAFF Manual of Nutrition* (available through HMSO) or the *Collins Gem Calorie Counter*.

To calculate the percentage of energy from carbohydrate, fat and protein, consult the box below, and compare with the recommendations.

To calculate % energy

$$\% \text{ Carbohydrate} = \frac{\text{g carbohydrate} \times 4}{\text{total calories}} \times 100\%$$

Recommendation = 60—70%

$$\% \text{ Fat} = \frac{\text{g fat} \times 9}{\text{total calories}} \times 100\%$$

Recommendation = 15—25%

$$\% \text{ Protein} = \frac{\text{g protein} \times 4}{\text{total calories}} \times 100\%$$

Recommendation = 15—25%

Modest reduction in calories

To lose 1 lb of fat per week, you need to have a calorie deficit of 3500 kcal per week, or approximately 500 per day. The most effective way of achieving this is by increasing energy expenditure and decreasing

Sample food diary

Time	Where	With whom	Food/drink	Quantity
7.30 am	Kitchen	Alone	Orange juice	1 glass
			Toast (white)	2 slices
			Butter	2 tsp
			Marmalade	4 tsp
			Tea with semi skimmed milk	1 cup
11 am	Office	Friends	Coffee with semi skimmed milk	1 large mug
			Doughnut	1
1 pm	Pub	Friends	Ploughman's:	
			French bread	6" piece
			Butter	2 pats
			Cheese	approx. 3 oz
			Coleslaw	2 tbsp
			Pickle	1 tbsp
			Lager	1 pint
6 pm	Kitchen	Alone	Digestive biscuits	4
			Coffee with semi skimmed milk	1 mug
7.30 pm	Dining room	Family	Fried sausages	2 small
			Chips	8 oz
			Peas	2 tbsp
			Lager	1 pint
			Ice cream	2 scoops
9.30 pm	Lounge	Husband	Coffee with semi skimmed milk	1 cup
			Chocolates	3 oz
			Baileys	2 glasses
Exercise	Walked to tube station – 10 min Walked to pub – 5 min Walked from tube station – 10 min Aerobics class – 45 min			

energy intake. So, for example, you could reduce your calorie intake by 300 kcal a day and increase energy expenditure by 200 kcal (a 45-minute walk). This is equivalent to a 500 kcal deficit per day.

If fat loss slows down or plateaus, reduce your calorie intake slightly further or increase the intensity, frequency or duration of your exercise programme.

◆ *Low-calorie dieting and stress* ◆

Low-calorie dieting can lead to an increase in the production of the stress hormone, *cortisol*. Combined with intense exercise, cortisol can increase the loss of lean body mass by stimulating protein oxidation. Cortisol also reduces testosterone production, signalling the body to reduce anabolic processes and store fat. Therefore, to minimise lean tissue breakdown, it is important to avoid a drastic calorie reduction.

Never consume fewer calories than your BMR

Calorie intake should never be less than your basal metabolic rate (*see* box below), otherwise you risk losing excessive lean tissue, severely depleting your glycogen stores and having an inadequate nutrient intake. In practice, most trainers should be able to lose weight eating 1500—2000 kcal per day, especially if they increase their activity level. It is erroneous and potentially dangerous to prescribe low-calorie diets of 1000 kcal or less.

How to estimate your BMR

Men		Women	
Weight (kg)	*BMR (kcal/day)*	*Weight (kg)*	*BMR (kcal/day)*
70	1680	50	1250
75	1730	55	1290
80	1790	60	1330
85	1850	65	1370
90	1910	70	1410
95	1960	75	1450
100	2020	80	1500

Trim the fat

Look carefully at your food diary and identify the high fat foods that you are currently eating. Aim to reduce intake to 15—25% by making lower fat substitutions – check the boxes below for suggestions. Remember, don't eliminate fat completely, as we need the equivalent of around 1 tbsp of oil (or 1 oz nuts or seeds) per day to get the necessary essential fatty acids and vitamin E.

No foods should be banned completely or regarded as taboo – this could lead to an obsessive and negative attitude towards food, which is psychologically harmful in the long term. All foods are allowable – it's the frequency and amounts that need watching!

◆ *Trim the fat I* ◆

Eat less of the following:

- ◆ butter, margarine and other spreading fats
- ◆ fried foods
- ◆ fatty meats and processed meat products (e.g. sausages, burgers, meat pies)
- ◆ pastry dishes
- ◆ cakes, biscuits, puddings
- ◆ chocolate
- ◆ crisps and similar potato/corn/wheat snacks.

(These foods are high in fat but relatively low in other essential nutrients.)

◆ *Trim the fat II* ◆

Make the following substitutions:

- ◆ semi skimmed or skimmed milk instead of full fat milk
- ◆ low fat spread or peanut butter instead of butter/margarine
- ◆ low fat/reduced fat cheese instead of ordinary cheese
- ◆ jacket potatoes, boiled potatoes instead of chips
- ◆ chicken, fish and lean meat instead of fatty meat, burgers and sausages
- ◆ crackers, rice cakes, fruit bars instead of biscuits and cakes
- ◆ fresh fruit instead of chocolate.

(These foods provide some fat together with other essential nutrients.)

83

◆ *Trim the fat III* ◆

Make the following changes:

◆ limit frying except stir frying, using only minimal amounts of oil
◆ top baked potatoes with fromage frais, yoghurt, half fat crème fraîche or baked beans
◆ remove skin from chicken or turkey
◆ grill, bake, stir fry or boil instead of frying
◆ make low fat salad dressings with flavoured vinegar (e.g. raspberry); yoghurt seasoned with fresh herbs, lemon or lime juice; fromage frais seasoned with mustard
◆ choose lean cuts of meat and trim off as much fat as possible.

(These will reduce your fat intake while supplying other essential nutrients.)

◆ *Low fat snack ideas* ◆

◆ Sandwiches, rolls, pitta, bagels with low fat fillings, e.g. banana, cottage cheese, tuna, chicken, salad
◆ English muffins, fruit buns, scones, potato scones/farls
◆ Breadsticks
◆ Oat pancakes, Scotch pancakes, homemade pancakes
◆ Oatcakes, wheat crackers and rice cakes with low fat toppings, e.g. banana, fruit spread
◆ Toast with honey/fruit spread/baked beans
◆ Fresh fruit, e.g. bananas, apples, pears, grapes
◆ Dried fruit, e.g. raisins, apricots, dates, apple rings
◆ Dried fruit bars, some cereal bars
◆ Home made shakes (low fat milk, fruit and yoghurt)
◆ Low fat yoghurt, fromage frais
◆ Baked potatoes with low fat fillings, e.g. fromage frais, cottage cheese, baked beans
◆ Breakfast cereals with low fat milk

Eat more frequently

Eat at least 4—6 times a day, planning snacks and meals at regular intervals. The advantages of this eating pattern include:

◆ an increased metabolic rate – dietary thermogenesis accounts for an approximate 10% increase in calorie expenditure following each meal

- steady blood sugar and insulin levels
- control of blood cholesterol levels
- efficient glycogen replenishment
- minimal fat deposition.

Make gradual lifestyle changes

A few changes in lifestyle are necessary to achieve long-term weight management. One of the biggest barriers is an unwillingness to commit to change. The box below lists some of the common reasons why many people fail to manage their weight in the long term together with some suggestions as to how to overcome them.

Lifestyle changes

Lifestyle 'Excuse'	Suggestion
Not enough time to prepare healthy meals	Plan meals in advance so all ingredients are at hand. Quick meals include baked potatoes, pasta with tomato sauce, beans on toast. Cook in bulk and refrigerate/freeze portions.
Work shifts	Plan regular snack breaks and take your own food with you.
Work involves lots of travelling	Take portable snacks, e.g. rolls, fruit, energy bars, muffins, dried fruit, fruit juice (diluted).
Need to cook for rest of family	Adapt favourite family meals, e.g. spaghetti bolognese, to contain less fat, more carbohydrate and fibre (e.g. leaner mince, more vegetables, wholemeal pasta). Make meals that everyone enjoys.
Overeat when stressed	Consider stress counselling or relaxation courses; learn to handle stressful situations; take up new sport/hobby/leisure interests.
Eat out frequently	Choose lower fat, higher carbo-hydrate meals in restaurants, e.g. pasta with tomato sauces, chicken tikka with chappati, stir fried vegetables with rice.

All calories are not equal

You need to have a negative energy balance to lose weight. However, new research suggests that the relative amount of fat, carbohydrate and protein in your diet is more important than the total calories.

Protein and carbohydrate calories

When proteins or carbohydrates are consumed, they cause an increase in protein/carbohydrate oxidation, thus increasing the body's metabolic rate. A significant proportion of protein or carbohydrate calories are therefore given off as heat.

In practice it is relatively difficult for the body to convert surplus protein or carbohydrate calories into fat as it is an energetically wasteful process. They are stored as glycogen, and only if they are eaten excessively will they be converted into fat.

Fat calories

Dietary fat is far more likely to make you put on weight than any other nutrient. Any fat eaten that is not required immediately is stored as adipose (fat) tissue; however, unlike protein and carbohydrate, fat consumption does not increase fat oxidation. Fat also contains more than double the calories per gram (9 kcal/g) compared with carbohydrate and protein (both 4 kcal/g).

It is easy to overeat fat calories for two reasons. Firstly, fatty foods usually have a high calorie density and low bulk, so it is easier to overeat fat calories than carbohydrate or protein calories without feeling full. Secondly, studies have shown that fat is not as satiating as other nutrients – it is not digested and absorbed as rapidly after meals as carbohydrate or protein, and while carbohydrate produces a rise in blood glucose, fat often depresses blood glucose, which means carbohydrate produces more rapid satiety than fat.

A low fat, high carbohydrate diet is the cornerstone of long-term successful weight control. If you eat until your appetite is satisfied and stick to low fat foods, body fat levels will automatically be controlled.

Dieting and metabolic rate

Studies have shown that basal metabolic rate is proportional to total body weight – the heavier you are, the higher your BMR. The proportion of lean mass to fat mass also has a small effect on BMR. Lean tissue is active tissue and burns more energy than fat (both at rest and during exercise). Thus, if two people weigh the same but one has a higher amount of lean tissue and less fat, they will have a slightly higher BMR than the other person. However, this makes only a relatively small difference to BMR since fat mass also has an additional energy cost, i.e. extra energy is used to support the fat mass.

BMR can be predicted from total body weight using standard equations developed by the World Health Organisation (*see* box below).

◆ *Finding your total daily expenditure* ◆ *(the number of calories to maintain your weight)*	
1. Inactive people	(very inactive occupation; sitting most of the day; no sport/exercise) = **1.3 x BMR**
2. Moderately active people	(inactive occupation; light activity at home; occasional sport/exercise) = **1.5 x BMR**
3. Active people	(active occupation or regular strenuous exercise/sport or daily walking/cycling) = **1.7 x BMR**

It is a myth that overweight people have a slow metabolic rate (except in rare cases such as hypothyroidism and Cushing's Syndrome), or that dieting slows your metabolism in the long term. When you restrict your food intake, your BMR falls initially (by about 10%) in an attempt to conserve energy, but soon returns to its original level after 1—2 weeks or once normal eating is resumed. To minimise the BMR reduction:

◆ reduce your calorie intake as modestly and gradually as possible
◆ perform regular aerobic exercise. This increases your energy expenditure and causes a short-term rise in BMR, the so-called 'afterburn' or 'excess post-exercise oxygen consumption' (EPOC)
◆ perform regular weight training – this increases lean body tissue, which is calorie burning tissue.

For example, if you normally eat 2500 kcal/day, cut down to between 2000 kcal and 2250 kcal and increase your energy expenditure by around 250 kcal per day. This will result in a calorie deficit of 3500—4750 per week, equivalent to a fat loss of 1—1.5 lbs per week. If your weight loss slows, you can gradually cut down to 1750 or increase your energy output. That way you will avoid or at least minimise a drop in your BMR.

Yo-yo dieting

Repeated weight loss and gain can result in altered body composition as lean tissue decreases with each 'diet' and fat tissue increases with each weight gain episode. In addition, fat tends to be re-deposited intra-abdominally, closer to the liver, rather than in the peripheral regions of the body, thus posing a greater heart disease risk. Repeated severe dieting can lead to a loss of lean tissue (including organ tissue) and nutritional deficiencies that can damage heart muscle.

Although there is no strong evidence linking yo-yo dieting with heart disease, it can also be bad for your morale and psychological health. Each time you regain weight, you experience a sense of failure which can lead to lowered confidence and self esteem.

Preparing for competitions

Competitive bodybuilding requires a very lean, defined physique with a body fat percentage considerably below the average genetic set range – males often attain a body fat percentage of between 4—7%, females between 10—15%. Some events have weight categories; others either have height categories or just a single class. If you are taking part in a weight-matched competition, it is an advantage to be as close as possible to the upper limit of your weight category.

Whatever the situation, your preparation will involve reducing your body fat level to increase your muscle definition. However, this should not be achieved at the risk of losing lean tissue (by rapid severe dieting), depleting your glycogen stores (by starving) or becoming dehydrated (by restricting fluids, or using saunas, sweat suits or diuretics).

The principles for competition preparation

Keep off-season weight close to competitive weight
The difference between your competitive and off-season weight should be no more than approximately 2 stone for men or 1 stone for women. If necessary, gradually reduce your body fat during the off-season so that you have less to lose pre-contest.

Allow enough time
In your pre-competition period, aim to lose a maximum of 1—2 lbs body fat per week; if weight loss is any faster you may be losing muscle mass. For example, to lose 1 stone (14 lbs) allow a minimum of 7 weeks, but ideally 14 weeks. Most bodybuilders allow around 12—14 weeks for their pre-contest diet preparation.

Monitor your weight and body composition
The mirror is usually the best guide to your progress. After all, your physique will be judged by its subjective appearance, not by body fat or muscle measurements. If you prefer to include objective measurements in your pre-competition preparation, you can monitor body fat by skinfold thickness measurements, girth (circumference) measurements, bioelectrical impedence or underwater weighing (*see* page 79).

Cut calories gradually
Estimate your normal off-season calorie intake, i.e. the amount of energy needed to maintain your weight, then reduce your calorie intake by a maximum of 250—500 kcal per day. If fat loss slows down, reduce your intake by a further 250 kcal per day but never eat fewer calories than your basal metabolic rate.

Increase aerobic training
Increase the amount and frequency of aerobic training. This will increase your calorie output while you are exercising and for a short

while afterwards (excess post-exercise oxygen consumption), thus speeding up fat loss as well as increasing the efficiency of your fat metabolism.

Carbohydrate intake = 60—70% of calories

Eat a high carbohydrate diet to maintain high glycogen levels. This will allow you to continue training hard, and help to spare muscle protein. If you do not eat enough carbohydrate, glycogen stores become depleted which increases protein (muscle) breakdown.

Fat intake = 15—25% of calories

Reduce your fat intake by avoiding fatty foods, cooking with less oil, and substituting high fat foods with low fat equivalents.

Protein intake = 15—25% of calories

Maintain (or increase) your protein intake to 1.4—1.7 g/kg/day. This will help preserve muscle mass and avoid protein breakdown.

Eat at frequent regular intervals

Divide your food into five or six equal-sized meals or snacks a day. This will encourage efficient glycogen re-fuelling, maintain steady blood sugar and insulin levels and ensure a constant supply of nutrients to muscle cells for growth and repair.

Rapid weight loss methods

Avoid having to lose weight at the last minute through starvation or dehydration as this can be dangerous and you will most certainly not compete at your best. Starvation leads to depleted glycogen stores and feelings of fatigue and lethargy, and also increases the loss of muscle proteins so muscle mass decreases.

Dehydration leads to electrolyte disturbances, cramp and heart-beat irregularities. It is doubtful whether you can re-fuel and re-hydrate sufficiently between the weigh-in and your competition so aim to be within your weight category at least a day before the weigh-in.

Pre-contest week

The main aims during the week before the contest are:

◆ to increase muscle glycogen levels which in turn increases muscle size and improves appearance

♦ to reduce water retention and therefore improve muscle definition and appearance
♦ to maintain muscle mass.

The best way to achieve maximum muscle glycogen levels is by
gradually tapering your training and increasing your carbohydrate
intake during the final week. Your total calorie intake should
remain the same as usual but the balance of carbohydrate : fat :
protein will change. Eat larger amounts of carbohydrate-rich foods
(e.g. potatoes, bread, rice, fruit, carbohydrate drinks) and smaller
amounts of fats and proteins. Ideally, your carbohydrate intake
should be 60—70% of energy.

The original method of carbohydrate loading – three days of
glycogen depletion through exhaustive exercise and a low carbohydrate diet, followed by three days of glycogen loading – has a
number of drawbacks. The depletion phase can leave you feeling
weak and drained and you may not succeed in loading sufficiently
over the next three days.

Recent research has found that you can achieve equally good
results by omitting the depletion phase, tapering training and gradually increasing your carbohydrate intake over seven days, a method
which can increase muscle glycogen stores by up to 30—40%.

Excess fluid can be eliminated by reducing the sodium content of
your diet to a minimum during the final three days. Avoid all
processed foods containing salt, such as tinned soups, sauces,
ketchup, and tuna in brine, as well as less obvious foods such as
bread, cheese and breakfast cereals. Low sodium sources of carbohydrate which can be eaten during the pre-contest week include:
rice; pasta; grains, e.g. cous cous, barley, cornmeal; sweetcorn; rice
cakes; potatoes, sweet potatoes, yams, plantains; oats and porridge;
fresh fruit, e.g. bananas, apples; dried fruit.

Carbohydrate loading

Taper training>>>>>>>>>>>>>>>>>>>>>>>>>Rest>>>>>>Competition

1	2	3	4	5	6	7

Increase carbohydrate intake>>>>>>>>>>>>>>>>>>>>>>>Competition

You should also increase your intake of potassium-rich foods to
help eliminate excess fluid and create a favourable electrolyte/fluid

balance. Suitable foods include fresh fruit (especially bananas, grapes, oranges and apples), vegetables, pulses and whole grains.

It is a myth that dehydration improves muscle definition. Electrolyte and fluid balance is regulated by sodium and potassium intake, not by water intake.

Contest day

Have a small, high carbohydrate meal or snack 2—3 hours before the contest. This will allow enough time for your stomach to empty sufficiently and for blood sugar and insulin levels to normalise before your event. Nerves can slow your digestion rate however, so you may need to leave a little longer than usual between eating and competing.

Choose foods which are familiar and agree with your digestive system, i.e. they can be digested and absorbed relatively quickly, and which are high in carbohydrate, low in fat and moderately low in fibre. More sodium can be eaten as it will not re-adjust electrolyte balance or cause water retention for several hours. Suitable examples include:

- ◆ porridge or breakfast cereal with low fat milk
- ◆ toast, bread with jam/fruit spread/honey
- ◆ sandwiches or rolls with banana/honey/jam
- ◆ pasta or rice
- ◆ rice cakes with banana or fruit spread
- ◆ baked potato
- ◆ fruit, e.g. bananas, oranges, grapes
- ◆ energy bars
- ◆ carbohydrate-based drinks/diluted fruit juice.

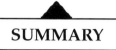

SUMMARY

- Keep a food diary for a week, listing the weight of everything you eat and drink. This helps you to become aware of your true eating pattern.
- Plan regular meals and snacks throughout the day, thereby eliminating excessive hunger, satisfying appetite, facilitating efficient glycogen re-fuelling and improving energy levels and health.
- Set yourself a realistic weight goal that is right for your body type.
- Do not set yourself rigid eating and exercising rules. Be flexible and never feel guilty if you overindulge or miss an exercise session.
- Examine your feelings and emotions when you eat. Food should not be used as a shield for emotional problems. Solve these with the help of a trained counsellor or an eating disorder specialist.
- The most effective way to lose fat is through a combination of reduced energy intake and increased exercise. The dietary strategy should aim to maintain carbohydrate and protein intake and reduce fat intake.
- Calorie intake should be reduced modestly and gradually to achieve a calorie deficit of approximately 3500 kcal per week or 500 kcal a day. It should not go below the basal metabolic rate.
- Rapid or prolonged dieting can result in loss of lean tissue mass and reduced metabolic rate.
- Overconsuming calories from carbohydrate or protein stimulates oxidation of these fuels respectively and they are less likely to be stored as fat. By contrast, overconsumption of fat does not increase fat oxidation and excess fat calories are deposited as body fat.
- BMR is proportional to total body weight and, to a smaller extent, lean body mass.
- Competitive athletes and bodybuilders should keep their off-season weight close to their competitive weight and aim to lose fat gradually within a realistic time frame.
- Rapid weight loss methods such as dehydration and starvation result in glycogen depletion, electrolyte imbalances, fatigue and poor performance.

Weight management (2): weight gain programme

Nutrition is equally as important as physical training when it comes to achieving significant strength and mass gains. Time spent in the gym each week could be wasted if you do not eat correctly.

The most common problem with strength training is very slow progress despite strict, strenuous training. The most common reason for this is a failure to eat correctly. Many athletes simply do not eat enough calories to support their training programme, while others (mostly men) are victims of dietary myths such as over-consumption of protein and a reliance on supplements.

Lean weight gain can only be achieved through a combination of a strength training programme and a balanced diet. Strength (resistance) training provides the stimulus for muscle growth while your diet provides the correct amount of energy (calories) and nutrients to enable your muscles to grow at the optimal rate. One without the other will result in minimal lean weight gain.

How much weight can I expect to gain?

The amount of lean weight you can expect to gain depends on three main factors:

◆ genetics
◆ body type
◆ hormonal balance.

Genetics

Your genetics determine the proportion of different types of fibre in your muscles. The fast twitch fibres are the power-generating fibres which increase in size more readily than the slow twitch fibres. So, if you naturally have a high proportion of fast twitch fibres in your muscles, you will probably respond faster to a strength training programme than someone who has a higher proportion of slow twitch fibres. Unfortunately, you cannot convert slow twitch fibres into fast twitch fibres, which is why certain people are naturally slow gainers and certain people fast gainers. Two people may follow exactly the same training programme, yet the one with many fast twitch muscle fibres will gain weight faster than the other.

Body type

Your natural body type also affects how fast you gain lean weight. An ectomorph – naturally slim build with long lean limbs, narrow shoulders and hips – will find it harder to gain weight than a meso-morph – muscular athletic build with wide shoulders and narrow hips – who tends to gain muscle readily. An endomorph – stocky, rounded build with wide shoulders and hips and an even distribu-tion of fat – gains both fat and muscle readily.

Hormonal balance

People with a higher natural level of the male (anabolic) sex hormones such as testosterone, will gain muscle faster than people with a lower level. That is why women in general cannot achieve the muscle mass or size of men unless they take anabolic steroids. However, everyone can still gain muscle and improve his or her shape with consistent training and good nutrition.

How fast can I expect to gain weight?

Muscle and strength gains are usually faster at the start of a strength programme and then gradually slow down. Gains are often periodic as each improvement is interspersed with a plateau.

As with a weight loss programme, aim to gain weight gradually. After an initial relatively fast gain, expect to gain up to 1—2 lbs per month or between 0.25—1% of your body weight per week. Monitor your body composition rather than simply your weight using a combination of skinfold thickness measurements and girth measurements. If you gain much more than 2 lbs per month on an established programme, you are likely to be gaining fat!

How much should I eat?

Research has found that in order to gain lean weight and muscle strength at the optimal rate you need to have a slight positive energy balance, i.e. consuming more calories than you need to maintain bodyweight. Undereating is the most common mistake that trainers (especially women) make.

If your weight has been relatively stable for several weeks, the best way to work out your optimal calorie need is to estimate your current calorie intake by keeping a food diary. Since it takes 2500 extra calories to gain 1 lb of muscle you need to increase your food intake appropriately. In practice, slow gainers should add an extra 500 kcal to their daily diet; fast gainers may need less (300—500 kcal). Not all of these extra calories are converted into muscle – some will be used for digestion and absorption, given off as heat (increased metabolism) or used for physical activity.

Protein needs

Studies have shown that the protein needs of strength trainers are greater than those of endurance trainers or sedentary people. Additional protein is needed to compensate for increased protein breakdown during training and to promote new growth and tissue repair.

Individual needs depend on three main factors.

(1) Training programme

Protein breakdown (catabolism) is increased during intense exercise. The greater the intensity, duration and frequency of your workouts, the greater the catabolism and therefore the greater your protein requirements.

(2) Training experience

With training, the body adapts to a lower protein intake. It becomes more efficient in re-using the amino acids released from the breakdown of proteins; in other words, fewer amino acids are lost through excretion and energy production so daily needs decrease. Experienced trainers therefore have a lower protein requirement per unit of body weight than beginners.

(3) Glycogen stores

High glycogen stores have a protein-sparing effect. When glycogen stores are low, protein breakdown increases to supply fuel for energy. If your carbohydrate intake is inadequate to meet your energy needs or when glycogen stores are severely depleted towards the end of a hard workout, you will break down extra protein and so your protein needs increase. On the other hand, if you maintain high glycogen levels by eating enough carbohydrate, protein breakdown will be minimised. Consuming small amounts of carbohydrate during intense training will also help offset glycogen depletion. In other words, protein will not be wasted for energy production and more will be available for tissue growth and repair.

Protein recommendations

Experts at the International Conference on Foods, Nutrition and Sports Performance (1991) recommended that athletes should consume between 1.2—1.7 g/kg protein per day. The lower end of the range (1.2—1.4 g/kg) is appropriate for endurance activities, while the upper end of the range (1.4—1.7 g/kg) is appropriate for strength and power activities.

So, for example, a strength trainer weighing 70 kg will need 98—119 g protein per day. However, contrary to popular belief, extra protein above the body's requirements is not converted into muscle.

In a study carried out at McMaster University, strength athletes were given either a low protein (0.86 g/kg), medium protein (1.4 g/kg) or high protein (2.4 g/kg) diet for 13 days. The low protein diet, similar to the recommended diet for sedentary people, caused the athletes to lose body protein (muscle mass). However, the medium and high protein diets resulted in an increased body protein content, i.e. an increase in muscle mass. However, no further gains were made by increasing their intake from 1.4 g to 2.4 g/kg.

Thus muscle mass gains do not increase in a linear fashion with increasing protein intake. Once an optimal intake has been reached, surplus protein is not converted into muscle.

The protein content of various foods

Food	Protein (g per portion)
Meat/fish/poultry	
Red meat (4 oz portion)	32
Chicken (6 oz portion)	38
White fish (6 oz portion)	30
Oily fish (6 oz portion)	30
Mince (4 oz)	25
Tinned tuna (4 oz)	25
Dairy products and eggs	
Milk (½ pint)	10
Cottage cheese (4 oz)	15
Fromage frais (4 oz)	8
Cheddar cheese (2 oz)	14
Yoghurt (1 carton)	8
Eggs (2)	14
Pulses and nuts	
Kidney beans (8 oz boiled)	15
Baked beans (½ large tin)	10
Lentils (8 oz boiled)	15
Nuts (2 oz)	13
Cereals	
Bread (2 slices)	6
Pasta (6 oz boiled)	5
Rice (6 oz boiled)	4
Other	
Tofu (4 oz)	9

How to meet your protein needs

It is not difficult to meet your protein needs from a balanced diet, as protein is found in a wide range of foods, including dairy products, meat, fish, soya, cereals, pulses, nuts and seeds (*see* box above).

However, only a proportion of the protein in food is absorbed and used for tissue growth. Proteins which consist of a balance of essential amino acids are generally well absorbed and utilised; those which are lacking in one or more essential amino acids are less well absorbed and utilised.

The usefulness of a particular protein is often measured by its *biological value* (BV) which indicates how closely matched the proportion of amino acids are in relation to the body's requirements. It is a measure of the percentage of protein that is retained by the body for use in growth and tissue maintenance. Egg white has a BV of 100 and therefore contains all the essential amino acids required by the body in closely matched proportions; virtually all of the food protein can thus be used for making new body proteins.

Other foods with a high BV (70—100) include dairy products, meat, fish, poultry and soya products. Plant foods such as cereals and pulses contain significant amounts of protein but are short of one or two essential amino acids (the *limiting* amino acids). These foods have a lower BV but eating a mixture of them is equally as good as eating proteins with a high BV. The shortfall of amino acids in one is complemented by higher amounts in the other, so the resulting intake increases the overall BV. This is called *protein complementation*. In other words, it is not essential to obtain your protein needs purely from high BV sources; a variety of both low and high BV protein foods is a healthy way to meet your requirements.

A few commercially produced proteins made from filtered whey (milk) protein have a BV greater than 100 as the balance of amino acids is specially altered in the laboratory to reflect the body's needs as closely as possible. These proteins are used in certain brands of protein supplements and meal replacements.

Examples of protein combinations which result in a higher BV include:

◆ porridge (cereal and milk)
◆ red kidney beans and rice (pulses and cereal)
◆ peanut butter sandwich (nuts and cereal)
◆ baked beans on toast (pulses and cereal)
◆ lentil soup with roll (pulses and cereal)
◆ chilli con carne (pulses and meat)
◆ breakfast cereal and milk (cereal and milk).

The BV content of various foods

Foods with a high BV	Foods with a low BV
Milk, cheese, yoghurt	Pulses – beans, lentils, peas
Meat, fish, poultry	Bread, cereals, grains
Eggs	Nuts and seeds
Soya products (soya beans/milk/ textured vegetable protein/tofu)	

Excess protein

Although strength athletes require a greater amount of protein in their diet than sedentary people, consuming more than you need certainly offers no advantage in terms of health or physical performance. Extra protein is not converted into muscle and does not cause further increases in muscle size, strength or stamina.

Research has shown that protein consumption increases protein oxidation in the body. In other words, when excess protein is eaten a quantity is used for energy and given off as heat. The amino part of the protein molecule is excreted in the urine while the remainder of the molecule is converted into glucose and used as an energy substrate. It may either be used as fuel immediately or stored, usually as glycogen. If you are already eating enough carbohydrate and therefore re-filling your glycogen stores adequately, excess glucose may be converted into fat.

Meal timing

Protein breakdown (catabolism) always exceeds assimilation (anabolism) immediately after training. At this point your body's priority is carbohydrate (glycogen) replenishment, not protein replenishment. Glycogen storage is faster during the two hours immediately following exercise and eating carbohydrate during this time therefore allows you to re-fuel and recover faster before your next workout (*see* pp. 66–7). Even if you finish training late in the evening, you should still have a high carbohydrate snack to start the re-fuelling process. Do not go to bed on an empty stomach after training!

Research also suggests that glycogen replenishment is increased by consuming small amounts of protein with high carbohydrate foods in the post-exercise period. Suitable snacks include sandwiches (filled with low fat cheese, tuna, chicken, peanut butter), cereal and low fat milk, pasta or baked potatoes with low fat cheese or fish, fruit and yoghurt or a commercial carbohydrate-protein drink.

Chapter 21 outlines eating plans which meet basic nutritional requirements and provide between 2000 and 4000 kcal. Follow a menu providing approximately 3000 kcal (*see* pp. 213–15) as a basis for developing your own daily menu.

◆ *Tips for hard gainers* ◆

- ◆ Increase your calorie intake by approximately 500 kcal/day.
- ◆ Aim for a gradual weight gain of 1—2 lbs per month.
- ◆ Eat at least 5—6 meals and snacks a day (every 2—3 hours).
- ◆ If you cannot eat large meals, include more snacks between meals.
- ◆ Include a mixture of high and low fibre foods in your diet so it is not too bulky and filling, e.g. wholemeal and white bread, fresh fruit and fruit juice.
- ◆ Some weight gain supplements may be useful for those with very high requirements who find it impossible to consume enough food.
- ◆ Obtain your extra calories from low bulk nutritious foods, e.g. dried fruit, milk-based drinks, yoghurt, fruit juice, energy bars and nuts rather than filling up on high calorie or fatty foods, e.g. biscuits, chocolate and cakes which are low in essential nutrients.

SUMMARY

- ◆ Lean weight gain is achieved through a combination of strength training (to provide the growth stimulus) and correct nutrition (to provide optimal nutrients and energy).
- ◆ The amount and rate of weight gain depends on genetics and hormonal balance. Your genetic make-up will influence body type and the distribution of muscle fibres.
- ◆ Most athletes will gain 1—2 lbs per month on an established programme.
- ◆ A slightly positive energy balance results in the fastest lean weight gain.
- ◆ Protein needs depend on the intensity, duration and frequency of the training programme, your training experience and size of your glycogen stores. An intake of between 1.4—1.7 g/kg body weight/day is recommended for strength training.
- ◆ Surplus protein is not converted into muscle and offers no advantage in terms of performance or health. It is converted into an energy substrate and stored as glycogen or fat.
- ◆ Protein needs can be fully met by consuming a variety of foods with a high and low biological value. Supplements are unnecessary, particularly if energy intake is adequate.

CHAPTER 10

Sports supplements

An increasing array of supplements promise to help you reach your training goals. They claim to increase muscle mass and strength and give you that extra training edge, but do they really work or are they nothing more than marketing hype? This chapter examines the scientific evidence behind the claims and considers whether supplements can actually benefit performance.

Protein-based supplements

Most protein drinks are based around powdered milk and/or egg protein (soya is also available), and may contain a source of carbohydrate such as glucose polymers, as well as amino acids, vitamins, minerals, herbal extracts and various plant substances claiming to increase growth.

Protein-based supplements contribute to your daily protein intake but do not automatically encourage muscle growth, strength or endurance. There is no special ingredient that gives you extra strength or size. Even the added 'growth promoting' substances (e.g. dibencozide, ferulic acid, chromium picolinate, wild yam, ginseng) have no proven benefit.

It is possible to fulfil your protein requirements adequately from food alone, providing that you plan your diet sensibly. One pint of milk (any type), for example, provides roughly the same amount of protein as one serving of a standard protein supplement, but for considerably less money!

The only case in which they may be useful is for those people with very high calorie and protein requirements who would otherwise find it difficult to eat enough food. As an addition to meals, they provide a convenient low-bulk way of consuming extra calories, protein, vitamins and minerals. It is best to choose a supplement which provides a good balance of nutrients, and to always consume the supplement in between meals, not in place of them.

Remember that extra protein over and above your requirements will not be turned into muscle!

Amino acid supplements

Many trainers believe that amino acid supplements increase their strength and muscle mass. Manufacturers claim that supplements are useful because they do not need to be digested and are therefore absorbed faster; however, there is no evidence to support this as it takes hours to build new muscle proteins! What's more, in terms of the amount of nitrogen retained in the body, there is no difference between amino acid supplements and proteins from food sources.

Free-form or singular amino acids were popular in the 1980s, but later studies have shown that short chains of two or three amino acids (*peptides*) are absorbed more efficiently than single amino acids.

Another claim is that a greater percentage of amino acids is absorbed from supplements than from food. In fact, more than 80—90% of amino acids from food are utilised by the body, and supplements provide only small amounts of amino acid relative to your total dietary needs. Most tablets/capsules contain a gram or less, whereas a tuna or cottage cheese sandwich provides around 20 g. Thus, relatively large amounts of supplement would need to be taken to have a significant impact on your daily amino acid intake – a very costly exercise.

'Growth hormone promoting' amino acid supplements

Certain combinations of amino acid supplements, for example *ornithine, arginine* and *lysine,* claim to increase the body's production of growth hormone (GH), which stimulates muscle growth and fat oxidation, and manufacturers instruct athletes to take them before sleeping and prior to training. This is not based on any valid scientific research, however. In the 1980s a handful of weak studies using high doses of arginine and ornithine or arginine alone claimed small changes in body composition and strength, but failed to measure GH concentrations. Another study meanwhile measured an increase in GH after arginine and lysine were given to growth-stunted teenagers, but failed to measure changes in body composition or performance.

In a study carried out at the University of Pittsburgh, eight male athletes completed two weight training sessions, one using supplements and one without. Both workouts produced an equal increase in growth hormone output; in other words, the supplements had no effect at all. In fact, exercise and sleep are natural promoters of growth hormone release, and there is no evidence at all that GH promoting amino acid supplements work.

'Branch chain' amino acid supplements

Branched amino acids include the three amino acids with a branched geometrical configuration: *leucine, valine* and *isoleucine.* They make up about 70% of muscle proteins and are broken down in increased quantities during intense prolonged exercise as glycogen becomes depleted. Some manufacturers claim that supplementing these particular amino acids before, during and after intense exercise may reduce or offset muscle protein breakdown; however, there is little evidence that supplements have a significant effect.

In a study carried out at the University of Limburg in 1994, 10 athletes were given either an electrolyte sports drink with added branched chain amino acids or the sports drink alone and were instructed to cycle to exhaustion. There was no difference in fatigue time and the researchers concluded that the branched chain amino acids had no effect on performance or endurance.

Weight gain or meal replacement supplements

Weight gain supplements are basically a mixture of sugar and/or glucose polymers (i.e. carbohydrate) and milk protein. Most also contain added vitamins, minerals, amino acids and other nutritional or herbal substances claimed to enhance muscle growth, with the aim of becoming a meal in their own right. Serving sizes are usually very large, in some cases providing an additional 3000—4000 calories per day.

They typically provide around 50—70% calories from carbohydrate, very little fat and most of the remainder from protein.

However, there is nothing intrinsically growth-enhancing in these products – they simply form a low-bulk way of consuming extra calories, carbohydrate and protein. For hard gainers who find it very difficult to eat enough food, these supplements may help make up their requirements, but for the majority of trainers they are an expensive way to meet your basic nutritional needs.

Some protein-based meal replacements contain an endless list of ingredients, including 'metabolic optimisers' and patented blends of amino acids and herb extracts, and claim to produce steroid-like effects. Their use is supported only by anecdotal evidence, however, and not by any firm research published in a recognised scientific journal. Those who say the product has 'worked' for them have most likely increased their calorie and nutritional intake by taking the product, and have followed a consistent training regime. Of course, equal gains can be achieved by a well-planned diet with ordinary foods.

Carbohydrate supplements

Carbohydrate (energy) supplements may be in the form of powders, ready-mixed drinks or bars. They are based on glucose polymers – man-made carbohydrates derived from the partial breakdown of corn starch, which consist of short chains of up to 20 sugar units.

The advantage of using glucose polymers instead of glucose or sucrose in a drink is that a higher concentration of carbohydrate can be achieved (usually between 10—20 g/100 ml) at a lower osmolality. That is because each molecule contains several glucose units yet still exerts the same osmotic pressure as one unit of glucose. So, it is possible to maintain isotonicity or hypotonicity with a relatively high carbohydrate content.

Also, glucose polymers are less sweet-tasting than simple sugars so you can achieve a fairly concentrated drink or energy bar without it tasting too sweet or sickly. In fact, most glucose polymer drinks and bars are fairly tasteless unless they have added artificial flavours or sweeteners.

Studies of glucose polymer drinks have shown that they can be beneficial during high-intensity exercise lasting more than 60—90 minutes. The reason is that they provide additional fuel and fluid, thus offsetting glycogen depletion and dehydration. For most strength workouts lasting one hour or less, dehydration and fuel depletion may be offset by ensuring adequate glycogen stores and hydration beforehand and drinking a hypotonic or isotonic sports drink (4—8% carbohydrate), e.g. diluted squash, fruit juice or a commercial drink. Carbohydrate supplements are unlikely to offer an additional benefit in this situation.

Carbohydrate supplements taken in liquid or solid form between meals may be helpful for trainers with very high carbohydrate (calorie) requirements who cannot consume enough food to meet their needs. However, it should be noted that most supplements simply provide carbohydrate and no other nutrients, so the rest of the diet would need to be packed with nutrients. The majority of trainers should be able to meet their carbohydrate needs from a normal diet consisting of complex and simple carbohydrates (i.e. potatoes, bread, cereals, pulses, dairy products and fruit).

Testosterone boosters

A number of supplements, mostly plant extracts, claim to boost the body's natural production of testosterone; however, none of these claims are supported by scientific evidence. One example is *boron*, for which support is based on a study carried out on boron-deficient post-menopausal women. More recent studies have shown boron to have no effect on blood testosterone levels, strength or body composition in healthy adults.

Plant sterols and herbal extracts such as *smilax, sarsparilla,* and *saw palmetto* also have no effect on testosterone levels and contrary to claims, do not boost lean mass or strength either.

Creatine

Creatine monohydrate is widely used by power and strength athletes to help them reach peak performance. It claims to sustain maximum power output for longer which, ultimately, means faster sprint times (for athletes and sports players) and bigger, stronger muscles (for weight trainers).

The supplement is available in powder and tablet form, and also as an ingredient in the new generation of bodybuilding meal replacements. Its use is based on scientific studies which show that creatine supplements boost the creatine content of muscle (by up to

30%), the phosphocreatine (PC) content by 20% and also improve performance. The greatest increases, however, occur in people who have low stores to start with, such as vegetarians who do not consume any meat or fish, the only dietary sources of creatine.

PC is a high energy compound; although it doesn't provide energy itself, it can regenerate ATP very quickly during anaerobic activity. Thus, high PC levels mean that more ATP can be produced and peak power output can be maintained for a greater length of time. In fact, PC is responsible for maintaining energy production during the first 30 seconds of high-intensity exercise.

Figure 5 *The inter-conversion of ADP and ATP*

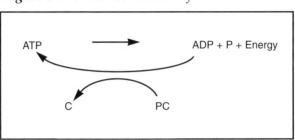

Studies have found that a dose of 20 g (4 x 5 g) creatine per day for five days results in maximal PC concentration in the muscles and produces an increase in performance of around 5%. Once saturated, the muscle creatine stores remain high for 6—8 weeks and can be maintained by a lower dose of 2 g per day. However, low dose supplementation without the initial dose will not improve performance. Higher initial doses have also not been shown to increase muscle creatine levels further.

Creatine supplementation benefits short-term explosive performance lasting between a few seconds and a few minutes. It appears to be most useful when repeated bursts of activity have to be performed with short recoveries (e.g. multiple sprints, sets of weight training exercises). In one study, seven male athletes completed five 6-second bursts of high-intensity stationary cycling (separated by 30-second recovery periods) before and after six days of creatine supplementation (20 g a day). After the five intervals, a further 10-second interval was completed. The ability to maintain peak power output in this final interval was enhanced after creatine supplementation. Also, lactic acid levels were lower (lactic acid limits exercise performance); however peak power output, as measured by jump squats, had not increased. This suggests that short-term creatine supplementation may enable you to train without fatigue at a higher intensity than usual.

Creatine itself doesn't actually increase strength but it can lead to faster training gains and, indirectly, improve strength and muscle mass. Indeed, several recent studies have found that creatine supplementation (20—30 g per day for five days) leads to significant gains in body weight ranging from 2—3½ lbs. Some of this is made up of water but some is likely to be lean mass. In one US study carried out by researchers at Experimental and Applied Sciences Laboratory, Texas Women's University and the University of Texas South-Western Medical Centre, creatine supplementation (20 g a day for 14 days) led to an increase in strength, total lifting volume (number of reps x weight lifted) and total and lean body mass. No significant changes were found in those taking a placebo.

Scientists believe that creatine increases lean mass by increasing muscle cell volume, shifting the amount of water that can be retained in a muscle cell. Increased cell volume is an anabolic signal to the muscle, causing it to take up amino acids and other nutrients. The result is increased muscle size, mass and strength.

Studies have found that you can maximise the effects of creatine if you mix it with a source of carbohydrate with a high glycaemic index, such as glucose, sucrose or fruit juice. The carbohydrate stimulates insulin secretion from the pancreas, which causes the muscle cells to take up yet more amino acids, glucose and creatine.

Glutamine

Glutamine supplements claim to be 'anti-catabolic', helping to stop muscle protein breakdown during intense training.

Glutamine is a non-essential amino acid that makes up more than half of the amino acid pool in the body and 5—7% of muscle proteins and, like other amino acids, it is broken down for energy during high-intensity exercise. It also plays a key role in the immune system. When immune demands are high, or during intense workouts or periods of stress, the body's glutamine requirements exceed production, and so muscle proteins break down to release glutamine. This leads to a state of catabolism (breakdown) and means that muscle growth slows down or stops altogether, despite hard training. Glutamine release is also greater when glycogen levels are low, e.g. when dieting or overtraining.

Glutamine supplementation may therefore offset muscle protein breakdown and conserve muscle tissue if you are undereating carbohydrate, training intensely or under stress. However, supplements are unlikely to have any effect if you are consuming adequate carbohydrates.

Vanadyl sulphate

Vanadyl sulphate claims to mimic insulin, thus increasing muscle growth and mass. So far it has only been researched with respect to diabetes. Researchers have shown that vanadyl supplements increased insulin sensitivity in people with non-insulin dependent diabetes, or allowed insulin-dependent diabetics to reduce their dose of injected insulin.

This supplement is also of interest to strength athletes as insulin is an anabolic hormone – it stimulates the uptake of glucose into muscle cells to make glycogen and also stimulates the uptake of amino acids into muscle cells to make new proteins. There is, however, no research to date on the effects of vanadyl sulphate on muscle strength or body composition although supplements have been marketed since the early 1990s.

Chromium

Chromium supplements claim to build muscle and reduce body fat. This is based on the findings of studies carried out in the 1980s which reported gains in lean mass and loss of fat in footballers and weightlifters; however, more recent studies have dismissed these findings and have found that chromium supplements do not alter body composition. The earlier studies have been discredited on the grounds of inaccurate body composition measurements.

Chromium makes up part of a molecule called glucose tolerance factor, needed for the regulation of insulin which, in turn, increases the uptake of glucose and amino acids by muscle cells. Low chromium levels (due to intense exercise or low dietary intake) can reduce the action of insulin, and supplements may correct a marginal deficiency but will not enhance muscle mass.

Carnitine

It is claimed that carnitine supplements speed up fat oxidation, conserve glycogen and increase endurance. Carnitine is found in meat protein but the majority is made in the body from two amino acids, *lysine* and *methionine*. It helps to transport fatty acids across the mitochondrial membrane into the mitochondria where they are broken down for energy. However, there is no evidence to support the claims for carnitine supplements. They do not increase fat burning – in fact, one study revealed that supplements increased glycogen breakdown!

Caffeine

Caffeine is a popular ergogenic (performance enhancing) drug used by athletes. It is a stimulant which, on the plus side, increases mental alertness, concentration and reduces physical and mental fatigue, but on the negative side can cause anxiety, nervousness, insomnia and dehydration (it is a diuretic).

The exact mechanism is not clear. It is likely that caffeine enhances fat oxidation, thus increasing the use of fatty acids for fuel and sparing glycogen, so fatigue is delayed. Another possible mechanism is that caffeine alters the body's electrolyte balance by retaining potassium in the muscle cells (fatigue occurs when potassium moves out of the cells). Caffeine may also have a direct effect on the nervous system or increase blood glucose concentration by stimulating glucose manufacture in the liver (*gluconeogenesis*).

Many studies have shown that caffeine can increase endurance and delay fatigue, but these have mainly focused on endurance events such as long distance running, cycling and swimming. Very few have been carried out on high-intensity exercise. One study at the University of Calgary in 1995 found that a caffeine intake of 6 mg/kg body weight improved swimming performance times in a 1500-metre trial. Those who consumed the caffeine drink swam significantly faster and experienced a lower perceived level of exertion. Thus caffeine improved performance, increased endurance and decreased athletes' perception of fatigue.

These results may also be applied to a weight training workout. It is feasible that caffeine may help trainers lift more weight, complete more reps or sets and decrease the perceived exertion by sparing glycogen. Relatively high doses of caffeine are needed to produce a performance enhancing effect. Most studies have used around 200—600 mg, equivalent to 2—6 cups of coffee, or alternatively have used caffeine tablets. It should be remembered that caffeine is a diuretic and also a banned substance above 12 ug/ml in urine (equivalent to 6—9 cups of coffee). It is your decision whether the negative effects outweigh the positive effects.

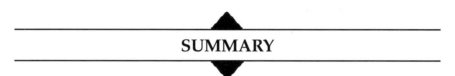

SUMMARY

- ◆ Weight gain and meal replacement supplements which provide a good balance of carbohydrate (60% energy), protein (15—25% energy), vitamins and minerals may be useful for meeting the nutritional and energy needs of hard gainers or those who cannot consume enough food. However, they will not automatically increase muscle growth.
- ◆ There is no evidence to support the use of amino acid supplements or specific amino acids claiming to promote the growth hormone.
- ◆ Carbohydrate drinks and bars based on glucose polymers may help to delay fatigue and maintain exercise intensity during high-intensity workouts lasting over an hour. For those lasting less than one hour or for moderate-intensity workouts, isotonic drinks containing 4—8% carbohydrate will provide enough fuel and fluid.
- ◆ There is no evidence to suggest that herb and plant extracts or plant sterols increase testosterone production, muscle mass or strength.
- ◆ An intake of 20 g of creatine per day for five days can increase muscle phosphocreatine (PC) levels and benefit high-intensity explosive activities such as weight training. High PC levels help maintain workout intensity and therefore produce faster gains in strength and mass.
- ◆ Glutamine may offset muscle protein breakdown but appears to be beneficial only when carbohydrate intake is inadequate.
- ◆ There is no direct evidence to suggest that vanadyl sulphate increases muscle strength or mass.
- ◆ There is limited evidence that caffeine improves performance during high-intensity exercise. Relatively high doses improve endurance and reduce the perception of fatigue; however, it is a diuretic and a banned substance over 12 ug/ml urine.

Stretching and warming up

It is important to warm up before beginning your training session for two main reasons: it reduces the chances of injury and will improve your performance.

Muscles respond better to exercise if they are properly prepared for the coming workload. Warming up increases blood flow to the muscles and lubricates the joints, allowing them to work more efficiently. At rest the muscles receive only about 15% of the total blood supply, but during exercise the requirement for fuel and oxygen sharply increases and they may need up to 80% of the total blood flow to meet the demand. Obviously, it takes time to re-route the blood and this cannot be achieved efficiently if you omit the warm-up and start exercising vigorously.

Warming up improves the elasticity of the muscles, enabling them to work harder, more efficiently and for longer before they fatigue. Warmth allows nerve impulses to be transmitted faster and makes the fluid surrounding the joints less viscous so the joint can move more smoothly.

Warming up also prepares you mentally for the work ahead; it increases arousal level and motivation. Performing one or two warm-up sets with light weights acts as a mental rehearsal and means that you can perform your subsequent heavier sets more effectively.

Before your weight training session, spend 5—15 minutes warming up. The time taken depends on the temperature of your surroundings – the cooler the environment, the longer it will take to raise your body temperature. The warm-up should include the following four components.

An aerobic activity that raises your body temperature and leaves you mildly sweating. This should be continuous and rhythmic in nature, for example, stationary cycling, treadmill walking, gentle jogging, stepping or rowing.

Mobilisation of the major joints This could include movements such as arm circles, knee bends and shoulder circles which take the joints through their full range of motion. These are not stretching exercises as they are continuous and do not increase the range of motion.

Stretching A few preparatory stretches relevant to the body part about to be exercised should be performed. These should be static (held still) rather than ballistic (bounced or forced) and maintained for at least six seconds. Muscles stretch more easily when they are warm and the muscle fibres are more pliable and elastic, so these stretches should be done towards the end of the warm-up.

Specific warm-up This concentrates on the muscles or body part you are about to use, for example, performing the first couple of sets of the exercise with very light weights. The effects are more localised, working the muscles and joints that are used in the main sets and rehearsing the action to be performed.

Why stretch?

Stretching before, during and after your workout serves three important functions:

◆ it helps reduce the chances of injury to muscles, tendons, ligaments and joint capsules
◆ it improves your performance
◆ it reduces post-exercise muscle soreness and speeds recovery.

Prior to a workout, stretching allows you to work your muscles over a fuller range of motion and so enhances the training stimulus. After a workout, stretching helps to eliminate the metabolic waste that accumulates during strenuous training so your recovery is faster. In general, stretching helps promote optimal functioning of the body's internal organs, the digestive system and the nervous system. It also releases endorphins, the body's natural painkillers which enhance mood.

How do muscles stretch?

The muscles contain receptors called muscle spindles which register information about the muscle's length and rate of change of length. One of their main jobs is to protect the muscles from injury, and so whenever there is a rapid change in muscle length, a reflex action is set up to shorten or contract it instead.

The muscle tendons also contain receptors called *golgi tendon organs* (GTOs) which register information about the degree of tension in the tendon. When a high force is registered, the golgi tendon organs enable the muscle to relax in an attempt to reduce the tension, thus acting as a safety mechanism for the muscles and tendons. If the intensity of a muscular contraction or stretch exceeds a certain critical point, an immediate reflex occurs to inhibit the contraction or stretch. As a result, the muscle instantly relaxes and the excessive tension is removed, and with it the possibility of injury. In other words, the GTOs shut down the muscle to prevent injury. If the GTOs did not exist, it would be possible to have a stretch or contraction so powerful that the muscle or tendon would be torn from its attachments!

Bouncing, uncontrolled or forced movements cause the greatest reflex response. Thus ballistic stretching can cause the muscle to contract and so increase the chance of injury. Static stretching which is carried out slowly and in a controlled manner will lead to a reflex relaxation of the muscle.

How to perform stretches

You should only stretch when your body is warm and the muscle is receiving an increased blood flow – stretching a cold muscle increases the risk of injury and reduces the effectiveness of the stretch. Therefore, you should only stretch towards the end of a warm-up, between sets or after a workout.

Static stretching is a far safer method of stretching a muscle than ballistic movements. Gradually ease into position as far as you comfortably can, and hold it, all the time focusing on relaxing the muscle. Stretch only as far as is comfortable and then hold that position. As the muscle relaxes, ease further into the stretch, gradually increasing the range of movement. Never hold your breath; exhale and relax as you go into the stretch. Never go past the point of discomfort or pain otherwise you could pull or tear the muscle/tendon.

Stretches should be held for a minimum of six seconds. These short stretches are sometimes called preparatory stretches as they are normally performed at the beginning of a workout. Developmental stretches, normally performed at the end of a workout or during a separate session, will produce longer lasting changes in flexibility and should be held for 30 seconds or more.

Ideally, stretching should be done not only before and after the workout but also in-between sets, serving as a kind of rest period.

How can stretching help enhance muscle size and shape?

It has been shown that incorporating stretching into a strength training programme leads to greater muscle growth, and enhancement of muscle shape and separation. Failing to stretch actually limits the growth rate.

When developmental stretching is combined with weight training it potentiates the effects of overload training. In fact, everyone, no matter what level, can benefit from stretching. Stretching elongates the *fascia*, a strong protective sheath of connective tissue covering all muscles and their cells, allowing the muscle underneath room in which to grow.

Fascial tissue can become thick and tough if the muscles are not stretched and are subject to a limited range of movement. The best time to stretch the fascia is when the muscles are very warm and 'pumped' (i.e. full of blood). This occurs during and after a workout, so stretch between and after sets.

Stretching is particularly good for muscle groups that don't respond well to regular training. It can help overcome plateaux and sticking points.

Strength through stretching is related to your golgi tendon reflex threshold, which limits a contraction well short of the point at which tendons would be injured. Stretching gives the muscles the ability to contract more efficiently without shutting down in response to stretched tendons. Obviously, it is desirable to have a high GTO reflex threshold, as this allows you to handle heavier weights and do more reps without the GTOs inhibiting muscle action. The higher the GTO threshold, the more intensely you can train, and the greater the gains in size and strength. Stretching your muscles regularly can help raise your GTO threshold. Some experts estimate that raising your GTO threshold can increase strength by up to 15—20%.

Stretching also increases flexibility, giving the muscles and joints a greater range of motion. It can prevent muscle soreness and promote faster recovery between workouts, and helps to release lactic acid from the muscle cells into the bloodstream so that it does not hinder further muscle contraction. Therefore, stretching during your workout may enable you to train harder and longer.

Stretching also improves posture and gives the body a more athletic or graceful appearance instead of that clumsy awkward gait that many bodybuilders develop.

Specific stretches

Basic rules

◆ Warm up before stretching – never stretch a cold muscle.
◆ Ease into a stretch gradually.
◆ Relax into the stretch.
◆ Hold the stretch for a minimum of six seconds.
◆ Stretch before and after your workout and, ideally, in-between sets.
◆ Breathe normally – do not hold your breath.
◆ Release from the stretch slowly.

Quad stretch (*see* page 117)

Hold onto a sturdy support with your right hand. Bend your left leg behind you and hold your left ankle. Keep your thighs level and press your hips forwards. Hold, then repeat with the other leg.

Seated inner thigh stretch (*see* page 117)

Sit on the floor and place the soles of your feet together. Hold onto your ankles and press your thighs down using your elbows. Keep your back straight.

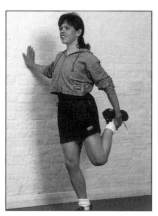

Quad stretch

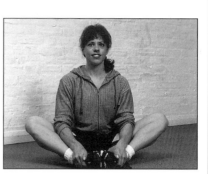

Seated inner thigh stretch

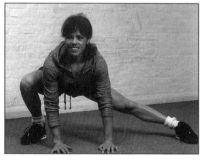

Standing inner thigh stretch

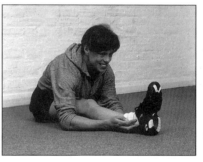

Sitting hamstring stretch

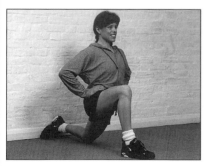

Hip flexor stretch

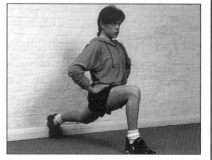

Gluteal, hamstring, quad stretch

117

Standing inner thigh stretch (*see* page 117)

Stand with your legs wide apart. Turn your right foot out to the side and keep your left foot pointing forwards. Bend your right knee and keep your left leg straight. Make sure your legs are wide enough apart so your right knee stops over your right foot. Either place your hands on your thighs for support or, for a more advanced stretch, bend forwards from the hips and place your hands on the floor. Make sure your knees are always in line with your feet. Hold, then repeat to the other side.

Sitting hamstring stretch (*see* page 117)

Sit on the floor with your right leg extended and your left leg bent. Keeping your back straight and flat, bend forwards from the hips. Reach down your right leg towards your foot as far as you comfortably can. Keep your head in line with your spine. Flexing your foot will increase the stretch on the calf. Hold, then repeat with the other leg.

Hip flexor stretch (*see* page 117)

Begin in a kneeling position. Take a large step forwards with your right leg so that your knee makes a 90-degree angle and is directly over your right foot. Keep your body upright and press your left hip forwards, keeping it square. You should feel a stretch across the front of your left hip. Hold, then repeat with the other leg.

Gluteal, hamstring, quad stretch (*see* page 117)

From a standing position, lunge forwards with your right leg so that your right knee makes a 90-degree angle and is positioned directly over your foot. Support your body weight with your hands on the floor to the inside of your right foot. Press your hips forwards and keep your back flat. Your left leg should be nearly straight. Hold, then repeat with the other leg.

Calf stretch (*see* page 120)

Stand with your feet hip-width apart, toes pointing straight ahead. Step forwards with your right foot, keeping your left leg straight. Make sure you take a big enough step so that your right knee makes a 90-degree angle and is positioned over your right foot. You should feel a good stretch in your left calf. Lean forwards slightly so that your left leg and body make a continuous line. Hold onto a wall for support if you wish. Hold, then repeat with the other leg.

Lat and side stretch (*see* page 120)

Stand with your feet shoulder-width apart. Raise your right arm overhead and bend over to the left. Place your left hand on the side of your thigh for support. Keep your hips level. Focus on reaching upwards and sideways. Hold, then repeat to the other side.

Lat stretch (*see* page 120)

Hold onto an upright support at waist height with your arms straight. Bend forwards from the hips until they make a 90-degree angle and your trunk is parallel to the floor. Gently pull back until you feel a stretch in your lats. Make sure you keep your back flat.

Upper back stretch (*see* page 120)

Stand with your feet hip-width apart. Clasp your hands in front of your body. Round your shoulders and curl your upper back forwards so you feel a stretch across your upper back.

Triceps stretch (*see* page 120)

Stand or sit upright. Place your right hand between your shoulder blades, hand pointing down and elbow pointing upwards. Use your left hand to gently press down your right elbow until you feel a stretch in the triceps. Hold, then repeat to the other side.

Shoulder stretch (*see* page 120)

Place your right arm across your body, elbow out and level with your shoulder. Gently press your right elbow towards the opposite shoulder. Hold, then repeat to the other side.

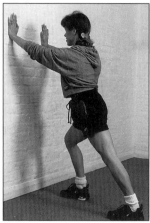

Calf stretch

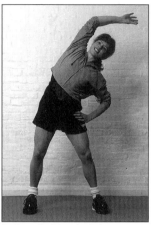

Lat and side stretch

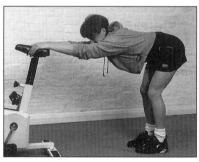

Lat stretch

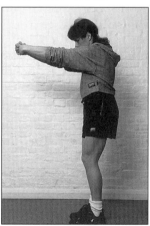

Upper back stretch

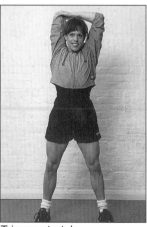

Triceps stretch

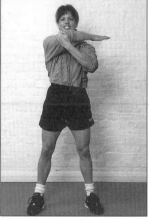

Shoulder stretch

Chest stretch (*see* below)

Stand with your feet hip-width apart. Clasp both hands behind your back, keeping your elbows slightly bent. Squeeze your shoulder blades together and pull your shoulders back. You should feel a stretch across your chest and the front of your shoulders.

One-arm chest stretch (*see* below)

With your right arm fully outstretched to the side, hold onto an upright support at shoulder level. Gently turn your body to the left, pressing your right shoulder forwards. You should feel a stretch across your chest and front shoulder. Hold, then repeat to the other side.

Biceps stretch (*see* below)

With your right arm fully outstretched to the side, hold onto an upright support at shoulder level. Flex your wrist back and gently lean away from your arm until you feel a stretch along the biceps. Hold, then repeat to the other side.

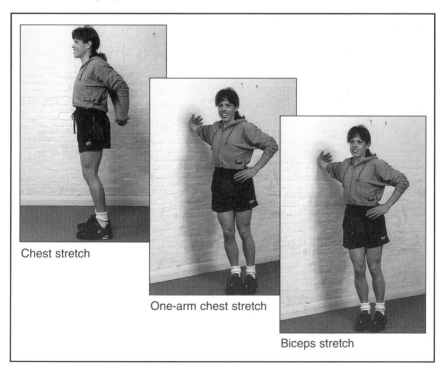

Chest stretch

One-arm chest stretch

Biceps stretch

Training technique tips

- Always warm up properly before starting your workout, making sure you include the four main components discussed in chapter 11: aerobic activity, mobilisation of the joints, stretching and exercise rehearsal.
- Select a suitable weight which will allow you to safely complete the desired number of repetitions. For mass and strength, aim to complete 6—10 repetitions; for muscular endurance, aim to complete more than 12.
- Perform each repetition using the entire range of movement, taking the muscle from its fully extended position to its fully contracted position.
- Avoid cheating movements as these will reduce the training stimulus and increase injury risk.
- Maintain full control of the weight throughout the movement.
- Hold the fully contracted position for a count of two before returning the weight to the starting position.
- Focus on both the concentric and eccentric phases of each movement. Resist the weight as you return it slowly to the starting position.
- The eccentric phase should take approximately twice as long to complete as the concentric phase.
- Rest for approximately 45 seconds—2 minutes between sets; the upper end of the range is more appropriate for heavier weights and exercises which use several large muscle groups.
- Ideally, stretch the worked muscles between sets.
- Perform longer (developmental) stretches immediately after the workout.

Why people fail to make progress

Choosing the wrong exercises

To increase muscle mass, you have to choose mass building or compound exercises (e.g. squats, shoulder press) which stimulate the largest muscles and the greatest proportion of fibres in those muscles. Choosing isolation exercises which work small muscle groups or only a small proportion of the muscle fibres in that muscle group will produce slow gains in mass.

Doing too many repetitions

Performing more than about 12 repetitions means that you are using a weight too light to stimulate growth in the fast twitch muscle fibres. More than 12 reps will improve muscular endurance and produce only small improvements in strength or mass. Therefore, if it is muscle growth you want, select a weight that will allow you to perform no more than 6—10 repetitions.

Doing too many sets

Research has established that less is best when it comes to building mass. You can achieve maximal stimulation of the muscle fibres by performing a strict set of 6—10 reps with a heavy weight to failure. Doing too many sets leads to glycogen depletion and increased protein breakdown, creating a net catabolic (breakdown) state, just the opposite of your goal! A maximum of 8—12 sets for a large muscle group and 4—8 sets for a small muscle group is recommended. If you can perform more sets than the recommended range, this means you have failed to train hard enough to fatigue the muscle and stimulate growth.

Not enough rest

If you don't give your body enough rest between workouts, you will not experience gains in mass or strength. One of the biggest mistakes made by beginners in their desire to make rapid gains is training too frequently. It is tempting to think that the more often you train the faster you will gain mass, but in fact the converse is true. Growth can only take place after compensation and full recovery. In other words, training before you have fully recovered can lead to protein breakdown and, over time, can lead to over-training.

Lack of progression

Many trainers become disheartened when strength gains slow down or plateau, despite maintaining a consistent workout programme. Indeed, it is easy to get stuck in a rut if you use the same weights, same exercises and same numbers of sets and reps. The muscles can soon adapt to a routine programme if the stimulus remains the same. In order to continue making strength and mass gains your training programme must be progressive, that is you must continue to increase the amount of stimulus applied. This may be achieved as follows:

- increase the number of reps (up to a maximum of 10—12 for strength)
- increase the number of sets (up to a maximum of 12 for major muscle groups and 8 for small muscle groups)
- change the type of exercises you perform and vary your workout, e.g. if you always perform lat pulldowns behind neck, seated rows and close grip chins for your back, change to wide grip chins, one-arm dumbbell rows and pullovers
- use different variations of exercises – different grip distances or feet positions, for example. Consult chapters 13 to 20 for new ideas
- change the order of your exercises
- change the training tempo, e.g. shorter rest periods between sets
- use different training techniques, e.g. slow rep sets, eccentric reps or supersets
- change the frequency of your workouts
- change the training split, e.g. train shoulders and back together instead of shoulders and arms.

Partial range of movement

If you use an incomplete range of movement, the muscle fibres receive only partial stimulation. You may be able to use a heavier weight doing partial reps but the overall stimulus applied will be greatly reduced. This is a very common fault made by trainers keen to increase the weight lifted – but it is at the expense of correct form.

You will achieve considerably greater gains by performing each repetition through the complete range of movement, even if it means using a lighter weight. Research has proved that taking a movement to the end of its natural range produces a more powerful anabolic stimulus than exercising over an incomplete range of movement. It also produces better muscle shape and prevents muscle shortening and reduced flexibility.

Poor technique

In an attempt to lift heavier weights, many trainers sacrifice technique. Not only does poor technique increase the risk of injury but it limits gains in strength and mass. 'Cheating' movements such as arching the back and bouncing the bar off the chest when performing a bench press, bending excessively forwards when squatting or swinging backwards when doing barbell curls, reduce the work done by the prime mover muscles and put the back at risk of injury. Correct technique is vital in order to make gains in strength and mass.

CHAPTER 13

Legs

The muscles

There are four parts (heads) to the front thigh muscle, known as the quadriceps – the rectus femoris, the vastus lateralis, the vastus medialis and the vastus intermedius – whose collective function is to extend (straighten) the knee. The rectus femoris also flexes the hip, i.e. lifts the upper leg up and forwards.

The vastus medialis runs along the inside of the thigh to the rectus femoris and can be seen on the inside of the knee when the leg is locked out; the vastus lateralis runs down the outside of the thigh and can be seen on the outside of the knee; the rectus femoris can be seen when the leg is lifted up and forwards slightly; while the vastus intermedius cannot be readily seen as it lies underneath the other muscles.

The main inner thigh muscles are comprised of three adductor muscles – adductor brevis, adductor longus and adductor magnus – whose function is to pull the legs together. The muscles of the outer thigh – the abductors – pull the legs out sideways.

The muscles at the back of the leg, the hamstrings, include the biceps femoris (long head), biceps femoris (short head), the semi-tendinosus, and semimembranosus. They have two main actions: to bend the knee and also pull the hip backwards.

Squats (*see* page 130)

Squats are an excellent all-round exercise for increasing mass, strength and power.

Muscles developed: gluteals, quadriceps, hamstrings, lower back, adductors, abductors.
To a lesser extent: calves, upper back, abdominals.

Starting position
- Stand erect with your feet shoulder-width apart, toes angled slightly outwards.
- Place the bar across the back of your shoulders.
- If you lack ankle flexibility and find it hard to balance while squatting, place your heels on a couple of small weight discs or a 1-inch piece of board.

The movement
- Keeping your head up and your trunk erect, slowly bend your legs and lower yourself down.
- Lower yourself until your thighs are parallel to the ground; do not go any further than this.
- Straighten your legs, pushing hard through your feet and keeping your body erect as you return to the starting position.

Tips
- Your knees should travel in the same direction as your toes – do not allow them to go inwards.
- Keep your rib cage lifted and your spine in a natural, slightly curved position.
- Keep your eyes fixed on a point in front of you at about eye level.
- Make sure you do not bend forwards excessively as this will strain your lower back.

Variations
Wide stance   Placing your feet just over shoulder-width apart with your feet angled strongly outwards emphasises the inner thigh muscles and gluteals. This is particularly useful for toning and building the inner thigh.

Parallel feet/narrow stance   Placing your feet parallel and a little less than shoulder-width apart emphasises the outer thigh muscles. This is particularly useful for developing the outer thigh.

Smith machine squats   Squats may be performed using a Smith machine. Since the bar travels in a straight line, there is less risk of lower back strain as you cannot lean forwards. Position your feet so that your heels are directly under the bar.

Dead lifts (*see* page 130)

Muscles developed: quadriceps, gluteals, hamstrings, hip flexors, lower back, latissimus dorsi, trapezius.

Starting position
♦ Stand in front of the barbell with your feet parallel and shoulder-width apart.
♦ Bend your legs until your hips and knees are at the same level, keeping your rib cage up and your head level. Your back should be straight, at a 45-degree angle to the floor.
♦ Grasp the bar with your hands just over shoulder-width apart, one facing forwards and one facing backwards. This will facilitate better balance and keep the barbell in the same plane.

The movement
♦ Using the power of your legs and hips, and keeping your arms straight, lift the bar from the floor until your legs are straight. The bar should be against the upper part of your thighs.
♦ Slowly return the bar to the floor, bending your legs and keeping your arms straight.

Tips
♦ Keep your back straight (i.e. in its normal position) throughout the movement.
♦ Keep the bar as close as possible to your body.
♦ Make sure your knees travel in line with your toes – do not allow them to travel inwards.
♦ Do not lean forwards – keep your weight through your heels.

Variations
On a block   Stand on a low, sturdy block or platform so that the bar is the same level as your feet. This increases the range of movement and, therefore, the benefits.

Incline leg presses

Muscles developed: gluteals, quadriceps.
To a lesser extent: hamstrings, calves.

Starting position
♦ Sit into the base of the leg press machine with your back firmly

against the padding.
◆ Position your feet parallel and hip-width apart on the platform.

The movement
◆ Release the safety bars and straighten your legs.
◆ Slowly bend your legs and lower the platform in a controlled fashion until your knees almost touch your chest.
◆ Return the platform to the starting position, pushing hard through your heels.

Tips
◆ Keep your back in full contact with the base; do not allow your lower spine to curl up as you lower the platform.
◆ Keep your knees in line with your toes.
◆ Do not 'snap out' or lock your knees as you straighten your legs back to the starting position.
◆ Make sure you do not bounce your knees off your chest.

Variations
Wide foot spacing   Placing your feet shoulder-width apart with your toes angled outwards puts more emphasis on the inner thigh muscles and will therefore help to develop this part of the thigh.

Feet higher on platform   Placing your feet higher on the platform so that your toes are almost off the edge puts more emphasis on the hamstrings and gluteals and will therefore help develop these muscles.

Leg extensions (*see* page 130)

Muscles developed: quadriceps.
To a lesser extent: anterior tibialis (shin).

Starting position
◆ Sit on the leg extension machine, adjusting it so that the back of your thighs are fully supported on the seat.
◆ Hook your feet under the roller pads.
◆ Hold onto the sides of the seat to help sustain your balance and keep your body upright.

The movement
◆ Slowly straighten your legs.

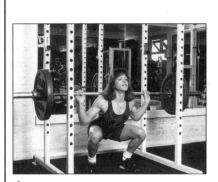

Squats

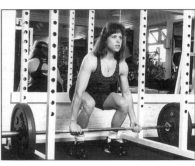

Dead lifts

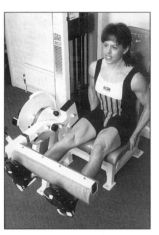

Leg extensions

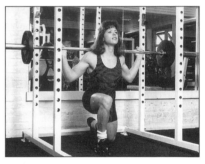

Front lunges

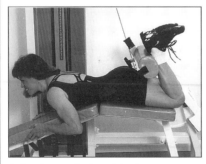

Lying leg curls (machine)

◆ Hold this fully contracted position for a count of two then slowly return to the starting point.

Tips
◆ Try to resist the weight back down to the starting point.
◆ Make sure you fully straighten the leg until the knees are locked.
◆ Avoid swinging/kicking your legs out straight – control the movement.
◆ Keep your thighs and backside fully in contact with the bench.

Variations
One-leg extensions   You can do leg extensions with one leg at a time. This allows you to concentrate fully on each repetition.

Toes outwards   Angling the feet slightly outwards places more emphasis on the vastus medialis, the thigh muscle that runs along the inside of the knee.

Toes inwards   Angling the feet slightly inwards places more emphasis on the vastus lateralis, the thigh muscle that runs along the outside of the knee.

Front lunges (*see* page 130)

Muscles developed: quadriceps, hamstrings, gluteals.

Starting position
◆ Place a bar across the back of your shoulders or hold a pair of dumbbells in your hands.
◆ Stand with your feet shoulder-width apart, toes pointing forwards.

The movement
◆ Step forwards with your right leg, bending the knee and lowering your hips.
◆ Lower yourself until your right thigh is parallel to the floor and your knee is at an angle of 90 degrees.
◆ Your left leg should be about 10—15 cm above the floor.
◆ Push hard with your right leg to return to the starting position.
◆ Repeat with alternate legs.

Tips
- ◆ Keep your front knee positioned directly over your ankle – do not allow it to extend further forwards.
- ◆ Keep your body erect throughout the movement – do not lean forwards.

Lying leg curls (machine) (*see* page 130)

Muscles developed: hamstrings.
To a lesser extent: gastrocnemius (calf).

Starting position
- ◆ Lie face down on the leg curl machine and hook your heels under the roller pads. Adjust the machine if necessary so that your knees are just off the end of the bench and your thighs are fully supported.
- ◆ Hold onto the hand grips or the edge of the bench.

The movement
- ◆ Bend your knees, bringing your heels towards your backside.
- ◆ Hold this fully contracted position for a count of two then slowly lower your heels back to the starting position.

Tips
- ◆ Keep your hips and thighs in contact with the bench throughout the movement – do not allow your hips to rise.
- ◆ Control the movement on both the upwards and downwards phase – avoid kicking your heels back fast.

Variations
Feet outwards Performing the movement with your feet angled outwards stresses the outer part of the hamstrings.

Feet inwards Performing the movement with your feet angled inwards stresses the inner part of the hamstrings.

Single leg curls You can do leg curls with one leg at a time. This allows you to concentrate fully on each repetition.

Lying leg curls (dumbbell)

Muscles developed: hamstrings.
To a lesser extent: gastrocnemius (calf).

Starting position
- Lie face down on a bench with your knees just off the end.
- Hold onto the edge of the bench.
- Bend your knees to 90 degrees so the bottom of your feet face the ceiling.
- Get your training partner to place a dumbbell securely between your feet.

The movement
- Slowly straighten your legs until almost parallel to the floor, lowering the dumbbell.
- Bend your knees, bringing your heels towards your backside.
- Hold this fully contracted position for a count of two then slowly lower your heels back to the starting position.

Tips
- Keep your hips and thighs in contact with the bench throughout the movement – do not allow your hips to rise.
- Keep your feet flexed throughout in order to hold the dumbbell securely.
- Perform the movement slowly, focusing carefully on your hamstrings.

Seated leg curls

Muscles developed: hamstrings.
To a lesser extent: gastrocnemius (calf).

Starting position
- Sit down on the leg curl machine and place your heels over the roller pads.
- Adjust the machine if necessary so that your knees are just off the end of the bench and the back of your thighs are fully supported on the bench.
- Hold onto the hand grips or the edge of the bench.

The movement

◆ Bend your knees, bringing your heels towards your backside.

◆ Hold this fully contracted position for a count of two then slowly straighten your legs back to the starting position.

Tips

◆ Keep your hips and thighs in contact with the bench throughout the movement – do not allow your backside to rise.

◆ Control the movement on both the upwards and downwards phase – avoid using momentum to perform the curl.

Variations

Feet outwards   Performing the movement with your feet angled outwards stresses the outer part of the hamstrings.

Feet inwards   Performing the movement with your feet angled inwards stresses the inner part of the hamstrings.

Single leg curls   You can do leg curls with one leg at a time. This allows you to concentrate more fully on each repetition.

Rear lunges

Muscles developed: gluteals, hamstrings, quadriceps.

Starting position

◆ Stand with your feet shoulder-width apart, toes pointing forwards.

◆ Place a bar across the back of your shoulders.

The movement

◆ Take a large step backwards with your right leg, bending your left leg, lowering your hips and keeping your trunk upright.

◆ Lower yourself until your left thigh is parallel to the floor and your left knee is at an angle of 90 degrees.

◆ Push hard with your left leg to return your right leg into position.

◆ Repeat using alternate legs.

Tips

◆ Keep your front knee positioned directly over your ankle – do not allow it to extend further forwards.

◆ Keep your body erect throughout the movement – do not lean forwards.

Cable kickbacks

Muscles developed: gluteals, hamstrings.

Starting position
- Attach an ankle strap to a low pulley machine.
- Stand facing the machine, about two feet away, and place your other foot on a small wooden block or weight disc.

The movement
- Extend your leg backwards as far as you can without twisting your hips.
- Return leg to starting position.
- Repeat with alternate legs.

Tips
- Keep your hips still and your legs as straight as possible.
- Squeeze your gluteals at the end of each movement.
- Keep your body upright – don't lean forwards.
- Don't use a heavy weight for this exercise – keep it light.

Symmetry problems

Skinny legs

Skinny legs produce an overall weak appearance. The symmetry problem is exacerbated if you have a well-developed upper body – a particularly common fault in men who put more emphasis on training their chest, shoulders and arms but neglect to train their legs!

The solution is to increase muscle mass in the leg area by concentrating on those exercises which cause maximum stress on the muscle fibres: squats, dead lifts and leg presses. These are, admittedly, harder to perform than isolation exercises such as leg extensions and curls as they require a great deal of physical and mental effort. However, they will produce faster and better results.

Symmetry programme for skinny legs

Exercise	Sets	Reps
Squats	1 (warm-up)	15—20
	3—5	6—10
Dead lifts	3—4	6—10
Leg presses	3—4	6—10

Straight hamstrings

The back of your thigh appears straight and flat when viewed from the side, as it is underdeveloped compared with the quadriceps. This imbalance is a common problem in long/middle distance cyclists and runners as these activities stress the quadriceps more than the hamstrings. It is also seen in weight trainers who have concentrated on exercising the quadriceps and neglected to balance their leg programme with hamstring exercises.

The imbalance can be corrected by cutting back on quadriceps isolation exercises such as leg extensions, and by including more exercises for the hamstrings, such as leg curls. Aim to increase the weight used and keep the reps in the 6—10 range. All-round mass builders such as squats and leg presses should still be included as they stimulate all the leg muscles equally.

Symmetry programme for straight hamstrings

Exercise	Sets	Reps
Squats or leg presses	1 (warm-up)	20
	3	8—15
Lying leg curls (machine or seated)	4	6—10
Seated leg curls	4	6—10

Wobbly thighs

Wobbly thighs or fat thighs are a combination of excess fat deposits (adipose tissue) and poor muscle tone. Lack of specific exercise leads to a gradual atrophy of the leg muscles, a decrease in strength and reduced muscle density. Eating more calories than you need over a period of time causes an increase in body fat stores. In women, this occurs mostly around the upper thighs and hips, thanks to higher levels of oestrogen, and is often referred to as cellulite (*see* page 20). It cannot be removed by creams, massage, body brushes or 'detox' supplements. The only way to reduce fat is to combine increased aerobic exercise with a lower calorie/fat diet.

Thus the solution for wobbly thighs is to include both strength and aerobic exercise in your programme, and reduce the fat content of your diet. Aim for a minimum of 20 minutes, 3—5 times a week, gradually increasing this to 45 minutes as you get fitter. Aim to train between 60—85% of your maximum heart rate.

The following exercises help tone your legs at the same time as burning fat:

◆ power walking
◆ jogging
◆ stair climbing (on step machines, stair masters or real steps)
◆ cycling (outdoors or using an indoor stationary bike)
◆ walking uphill or on an inclined treadmill.

Symmetry programme for wobbly thighs

Exercise	Sets	Reps
Squats or leg presses	1 (warm-up)	20
	3	12—15
Front lunges	3	12—15
Leg curls	3	12—15
Cable kickbacks	2	12—15

Shapeless legs

Although you may have good strength in your legs, they may lack shape. Viewed from the front, your legs make a straight line from the hips to the knees, with no obvious outer sweep to the thigh. From the side, your legs also look straight and neither the quadriceps nor hamstrings make an aesthetic arc. This makes your knees appear bigger than they actually are, a symmetry problem common among long distance runners and people who exercise regularly but relatively infrequently (e.g. once a week).

If you already have good basic strength and do not wish to build up your muscles much further, your programme should include isolation exercises such as lunges, extensions, curls and cable kickbacks. Squats and leg presses can be included less frequently, but use moderate weights and higher repetitions (15—25).

Symmetry programme for shapeless legs

Exercise	Sets	Reps
Squats or leg presses	2	15—25
Front lunges	2	12—15
Rear lunges	2	12—15
Leg curls (machine or seated)	2	12—15
Leg extensions	2	12—15

Gluteals

The muscles

There are three separate muscle groups, collectively known as the gluteals: gluteus maximus, gluteus medius and gluteus minimus.

The gluteus maximus is the largest, strongest muscle, largely responsible for the size and shape of our backside. It attaches to the lower vertebrae and the top of the rear part of the pelvis, and inserts on the top third of the back of the femur (thigh bone). Its function is to extend the hip in movements such as squatting, stair climbing and rear leg raises.

The gluteus medius is a smaller muscle, attaching at the top of the rear part of the pelvis and inserting at the top of the femur. Its function is to move the hip sideways (abduction) and also rotate the hip inwards, so it is used on the leg abductor machine or when doing leg raises to the side.

The gluteus minimus is the smallest of the three, attaching just below the gluteus medius and inserting at the top of the femur. It tends to act as a stabilising muscle, working eccentrically during impact movements such as running and jumping, and holding the hip joint in position.

Wide stance squats (*see* page 143)

Squats are an excellent all-round exercise for increasing mass, strength and power.

Muscles developed: gluteals, quadriceps, hamstrings, lower back, adductors, abductors.
To a lesser extent: calves, upper back, abdominals.

Starting position

◆ Stand with your feet just over shoulder-width apart, toes angled outwards at about 45 degrees.

◆ Place the bar a little lower down across your upper back than for standard squats. This is similar to the classic powerlifter's style.

◆ If you lack ankle flexibility and find it hard to balance while squatting, place your heels on a couple of small weight discs or a 1-inch piece of board.

The movement

◆ Keeping your head up and your trunk erect, slowly bend your legs and squat down.

◆ Lower yourself until your thighs are parallel to the ground – do not go any lower than this.

◆ Straighten your legs, pushing hard through your feet and keeping your body erect as you return to the starting position.

Tips

◆ Your knees should travel in the same direction as your toes – do not allow them to point inwards.

◆ Keep your rib cage lifted and your spine in a natural, slightly curved position.

◆ Stick your backside out behind you as if you are about to sit down on a chair (but don't lean forwards excessively), thus placing most of the stress on your gluteals.

◆ Squeeze and tense your gluteals as you push back up to the starting position.

Angled leg presses

Muscles developed: gluteals, quadriceps.
To a lesser extent: hamstrings, calves.

Starting position

◆ Sit into the leg press machine with your back firmly against the padded base.

◆ Position your feet high up on the platform, about shoulder-width apart, with your toes almost off the end and angled slightly outwards. This position places more emphasis on the gluteals.

The movement
- Release the safety bars and straighten your legs.
- Slowly bend your legs and lower the platform in a controlled fashion until your knees almost touch your chest.
- Raise the platform back up to the starting position, pushing hard through your heels.

Tips
- Keep your back in contact with the base – do not allow your lower spine to curl up as you lower the platform.
- Keep your knees in line with your toes
- Do not 'snap out' or lock your knees as you straighten your legs back to the starting position.
- Make sure you do not bounce your knees off your chest.

Rear lunges

Muscles developed: gluteals, hamstrings, quadriceps.

Starting position
- Place a bar across the back of your shoulders.
- Stand with your feet shoulder-width apart, toes pointing forwards.

The movement
- Take a large step backwards with your right leg, bending your left leg, lowering your hips and keeping your trunk upright.
- Lower yourself until your left thigh is parallel to the floor and your left knee is at an angle of 90 degrees.
- Push hard with your left leg to return your right leg to your original position.
- Repeat using alternate legs.

Tips
- Keep your front knee positioned directly over your ankle – do not allow it to extend further forwards.
- Keep your body erect throughout the movement – do not lean forwards.

Cable kickbacks

Muscles developed: gluteals, hamstrings.

Starting position
◆ Attach an ankle strap to a low pulley machine.
◆ Stand about two feet away, facing the machine, and place your other foot on a small wooden block or weight disc.

The movement
◆ Extend your leg backwards as far as you can without twisting your hips.
◆ Return the leg to its original position.
◆ Repeat using alternate legs.

Tips
◆ Keep your hips still and your legs as straight as possible.
◆ Squeeze your gluteals at the end of each movement.
◆ Keep your body upright – do not lean forwards.
◆ Don't use a heavy weight for this exercise – keep it light.

Rear leg raises on the floor (*see* page 143)

Starting position
◆ Begin the exercise on all fours, making sure your hands are beneath your shoulders and your knees beneath your hips.
◆ Extend one leg straight out behind you, allowing your toes to touch the floor.

The movement
◆ Raise the leg upwards, without moving your hips, until it is parallel to the floor.
◆ Squeeze your gluteals, then lower and repeat with the other leg.

Tips
◆ Keep your leg straight throughout the movement.
◆ Keep your hips still – do not allow them to twist.
◆ Keep your lower back flat.
◆ Wear ankle weights if you want to make the exercise more demanding.

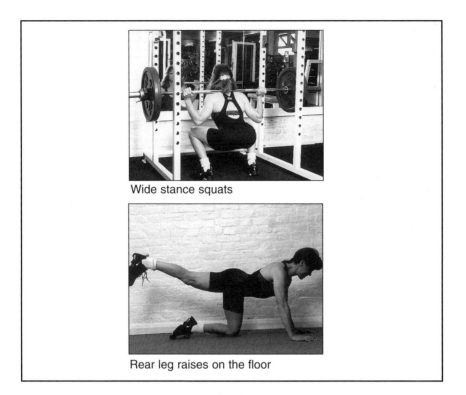

Wide stance squats

Rear leg raises on the floor

Symmetry problems

Large soft gluteals

This is probably the most common symmetry problem, due partly to the amount of fat covering the gluteals and partly to poor muscle tone. Fat accumulation is basically the result of overeating and lack of exercise over a period of time. In women, the female sex hormones favour fat deposition around the hips so it is possible to have a lean upper body but excess fat around the gluteals. It is also possible to have poorly-toned gluteals despite regular aerobic exercise, as many types of low-intensity aerobic exercise, such as walking and swimming, do not work the gluteals hard enough; the gluteals need direct exercise.

A two-way training and diet strategy may be necessary. To reduce the fat covering, include aerobic exercise in your programme for a minimum of 20 minutes, 3—5 times a week, gradually increasing to 45 minutes as you get fitter. Aim to train between 60—85% of your maximum heart rate.

The following activities help tone the gluteals at the same time as burning fat:

♦ power walking
♦ stair climbing (on step machines, stair masters or real steps)
♦ cycling (outdoors or using an indoor, stationary bike)
♦ rowing (outdoors or using an indoor machine)
♦ walking uphill or on an inclined treadmill.

Symmetry programme for large soft gluteals

Exercise	Sets	Reps
Wide stance barbell squats	1 (warm-up) 3	20 10—15
Rear lunges	3	10—15
Cable kickbacks/ Rear leg raises on the floor	3	10—15

For most effective fat reduction, combine your training prog-ramme with a low fat diet, following the guidelines on pp. 79—85.

Large overdeveloped gluteals

If you have overdeveloped gluteals, perhaps as the result of years of heavy squatting or power training, the only solution is to cut back on this type of exercise or at least to reduce the weight you use. The same applies to the other heavy power movements, such as leg presses and dead lifts – reduce the weight and increase the reps. Concentrate on other exercises which will work the legs but put less stress on the gluteals, such as leg extensions, front squats and leg curls.

Flat gluteals

Small, flat gluteals are due to underdevelopment of the muscles which tends to give a 'straight' appearance, particularly from the side, and also makes the waist look thicker than it actually is. The muscle group therefore needs to be developed, concentrating on heavy and basic movements such as squats and leg presses.

144

Symmetry programme for flat gluteals

Exercise	Sets	Reps
Wide stance barbell squats	1 (warm-up) 3—5	15 6—10
Leg presses	3—5	6—10

Droopy gluteals

Droopy gluteals are often the result of dieting without strength training; you have succeeded in losing fat from your hip region, but the underlying muscles are poorly-toned. The solution is to step up your calorie intake (in particular, carbohydrates and proteins) and include specific isolation exercises for your gluteals. Mass builders such as squats and leg presses may still be included in your routine, but you must use lighter weights and higher reps.

Symmetry programme for droopy gluteals

Exercise	Sets	Reps
Wide stance barbell squats or leg presses	3	15—20
Rear lunges	3	15—20
Cable kickbacks/ Rear leg raises on the floor	3	15—20

Back

The muscles

The major muscles in the upper back include the trapezius, the diamond-shaped muscle which extends from the back of the neck to the mid-back; the latissimus dorsi (lats), the large wing-like muscles that make up the majority of the muscle mass of the upper and mid-back; and the rhomboids, infraspinatus and teres muscles which are located around the shoulder blades.

Lateral pulldowns (behind the neck) (*see* page 147)

Muscles developed: latissimus dorsi, upper back muscles.
To a lesser extent: biceps, rear deltoids, forearms.

Starting position
◆ Hold the bar with your hands just over shoulder-width apart, palms facing forwards.
◆ Sit on the seat, adjusting it so that your knees fit under the roller pads. Your arms should be fully extended.

The movement
◆ Pull the bar down until it touches the back of your neck, simultaneously moving your head slightly forwards.
◆ Hold for a count of two then slowly return to the starting position.

Tips
◆ Keep your trunk as still as possible – avoid swinging forwards.
◆ Do not shorten the return phase of the movement – extend your arms fully.

◆ Return the bar slowly, resisting the weight on the return phase.
◆ Use wrist straps to improve your grip when using heavy weights.

Variations

Front of the neck   (*See* below.) This variation places extra emphasis on the anterior deltoids. Pull the bar down in front of the neck until it just touches the upper chest. Avoid swinging your body backwards.

Close grip   This variation thickens the latissimus dorsi rather than widening them, thus creating more depth to the mid-back. Use a triangle bar attachment and bring it down in front of your neck until it just touches the mid-point of your chest. Again, avoid swinging backwards.

Reverse grip   This variation also thickens the latissimus dorsi rather than widening them, thus creating more depth to the mid-back. Use a short straight bar attachment and hold the bar with your palms facing towards you about 6—9 inches apart.

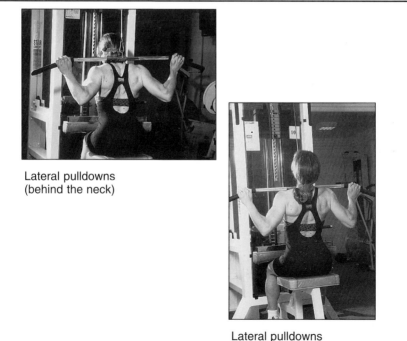

Lateral pulldowns
(behind the neck)

Lateral pulldowns
(front of the neck)

Chins (*see* page 151)

Muscles developed: latissimus dorsi, upper back muscles.
To a lesser extent: biceps, rear deltoids, forearms.

Starting position
◆ Hang from a chinning bar with your hands just over shoulder-width apart, palms facing forwards.
◆ Your arms should be fully extended and your ankles crossed.

The movement
◆ Pull yourself up slowly until the base of your neck just touches the bar. Lead with your upper chest.
◆ Pause for a second or two then slowly lower yourself back to the starting position.

Tips
◆ Do not swing your legs forwards or jerk as you pull yourself up – this reduces the stress placed on the back muscles.
◆ Fix your eyes slightly upwards as you pull yourself up, just arching your back.
◆ Ensure your trunk and thighs maintain a straight line.
◆ Do not shorten the return phase of the movement – extend your arms fully.

Variations
Behind neck   This variation places extra emphasis on the rhomboids (upper back muscles) and posterior deltoids. Pull yourself up until the base of your neck just touches the bar.

Close grip   This variation places more stress on the lower lats and biceps. Use either an overhand or underhand grip with your hands shoulder-width apart.

Parallel grip   This variation works the lower lats as well as the middle, adding thickness and density to these regions of the back. Hook a triangle bar over the chinning bar and pull yourself up so that your mid-chest touches the triangle bar.

One-arm rows (*see* page 151)

Muscles developed: latissimus dorsi, upper back muscles.
To a lesser extent: biceps, posterior deltoids.

Starting position
◆ Hold a dumbbell in your right hand.
◆ Bend forwards from the waist, placing your left hand and knee on a bench to stabilise yourself. Your back should be flat and almost horizontal and your right arm fully extended.

The movement
◆ Pull the dumbbell up towards your waist as you bend your elbow. Keep the dumbbell close to your body.
◆ Pause for a moment then slowly lower the dumbbell until your arm is fully extended.
◆ Repeat using alternate legs.

Tips
◆ Keep your lower back flat and still.
◆ Pull the dumbbell up slowly – do not jerk it up.

Seated cable rows (*see* page 151)

Muscles developed: latissimus dorsi, trapezius.
To a lesser extent: biceps, forearms.

Starting position
◆ Attach a short straight bar to the low pulley.
◆ Sit facing the cable row machine and place your feet against the stop bar. Grasp the bar and bend your knees slightly.

The movement
◆ Pull the bar towards you until it touches your lower rib/upper abdomen region.
◆ Hold for a count of two then slowly return to the starting position.

Tips
◆ Arch your back as you pull the bar towards you, keeping your chest out.
◆ Fully extend your arms as you return the bar, stretching forwards to achieve a good stretch on your lats.

◆ Do not lean or jerk backwards as you pull the bar towards you – your lower back should remain still.
◆ Keep your elbows close into your body.

Variations
Triangle bar   Cable rows may be performed using a triangle bar instead of a straight bar.

Dumbbell pullovers (*see* page 151)

Muscles developed: latissimus dorsi, pectorals.

Starting position
◆ Lie across a flat bench with your shoulders and upper back supported and your feet flat on the floor, shoulder-width apart.
◆ Hold a dumbbell with both hands, turned so that your palms are against the inside of one end plate.
◆ Hold the dumbbell above your chest with your arms extended.

The movement
◆ Slowly lower the dumbbell behind your head, keeping your arms almost straight, until your elbows are level with your ears and your hands are just beyond the top of your head.
◆ Allow your hips to drop down as you lower the dumbbell.
◆ Pull the dumbbell slowly back to the starting position.

Tips
◆ Do not allow your hips to rise up as you lower the dumbbell – drop them down.
◆ Inhale deeply as you lower the dumbbell and exhale as you return it to the starting position.
◆ Keep a slight bend in your elbows (10—15 degrees).

Dead lifts

Muscles developed: quadriceps, gluteals, hamstrings, hip flexors, lower back, latissimus dorsi, trapezius.

Starting position
◆ Stand in front of the barbell with your feet parallel and shoulder-width apart. Bend your legs, keeping your body erect, and head level.

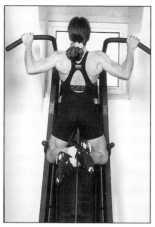

Chins

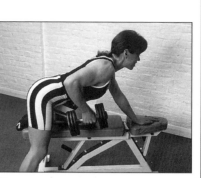

One-arm rows

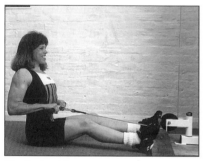

Seated cable rows

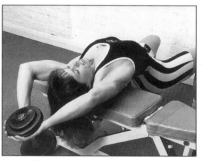

Dumbbell pullovers

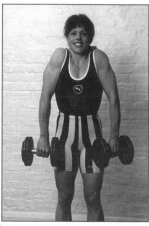

Shrugs

◆ Grasp the bar with your hands just over shoulder-width apart, one facing forwards and one facing backwards.

The movement
◆ Using the power of your legs and hips, and keeping your arms straight, lift the bar from the floor until your legs are straight. The bar should be resting against the upper part of your thighs.
◆ Slowly return the bar to the floor, bending your legs and keeping your arms straight.

Tips
◆ Keep your back straight throughout the movement.
◆ Keep the bar as close to your body as possible.
◆ Make sure your knees travel in line with your toes – do not allow them to travel inwards.
◆ Do not lean forwards – keep your weight through your heels.

Variations
On a block Stand on a low sturdy block or platform so that the bar is level with your feet. This increases the range of movement and, therefore, the benefits.

Shrugs (*see* page 151)

Muscles developed: trapezius, other neck and shoulder girdle muscles.

Starting position
◆ Stand with your feet hip-width apart.
◆ Hold a pair of dumbbells by your sides, level with your thighs, palms facing the rear. Keep your arms straight.

The movement
◆ Shrug your shoulders straight up, as high as possible, keeping your arms straight.
◆ Hold for a count of two then lower the dumbbells back to the starting position.

Tips
◆ Aim to touch your ears with your shoulders.
◆ Keep your shoulders back and your chest out.

- Keep your arms straight at all times.
- Lift and lower the dumbbells slowly and deliberately – don't jerk them up.
- As you lower the dumbbells, allow your shoulders to drop down as far as possible – this stretches the trapezius and increases the range of movement.
- Do not rotate your shoulders backwards at the top of the movement – this increases the risk of injury to the shoulder and places no further work on the trapezius.
- Use straps to improve your grip.

Variations
Barbell shrugs   Shrugs may be performed with a barbell, instead of dumbbells. Hold a barbell in front of or behind your thighs, keep your arms straight and move the bar up and down.

Hyperextensions

Muscles developed: spinal extensors.

Starting position
- Lie face down on the floor.
- Place your hands by the sides of your head, elbows out to the sides.

The movement
- Raise your head, shoulders and upper chest from the floor.
- Pause for a count of two then lower yourself slowly to the floor.

Tips
- Keep your head face downwards to the floor in line with your spine.
- Keep your legs relaxed on the floor – do not raise them.
- Only raise yourself as far as you feel comfortable.

Variations
Hyperextensions may be performed across a hyperextension bench. Hook your heels underneath the pads and position your body so that your hips are resting on the middle pad. Raise your torso until you are parallel with the floor – do not rise higher than this.

To make the movement easier, place your hands by your sides.

To make the movement harder, place your arms over your head by your ears; or, only if you are advanced, hold a small weight disc against your chest.

Symmetry problems

Narrow back

Viewed from behind, your torso is straight, narrow and lacks a pleasing 'V' taper. This is mainly due to the underdevelopment of the back muscles and is a very common problem, especially in people who do little exercise. It is also seen in long distance runners, joggers, cyclists, aerobics participants, and many other sportsmen since relatively few sports work this muscle group. Rowing, boxing and swimming (particularly the butterfly and crawl strokes) are good for developing the back muscles.

The solution is to build and develop the muscles of the upper and mid-back using basic power movements. The exercises in this programme build both width and thickness and will create a symmetrical 'V' taper to your back.

Symmetry programme for a narrow back

Exercise	Sets	Reps
Dead lifts	3	8—12
Chins (wide grip)	3	8—10 (or as many as possible, if less than 8)
Lat pulldowns (behind neck)	3	8—12
One-arm rows	3	8—12

Flat upper back

From the side, your upper back looks flat and thinly muscled. The back lacks thickness and density and the natural lumber curve is diminished. However, when viewed from behind, your back may have reasonably good width due to a naturally wide bone structure or to a limited amount of training which has built width but not thickness.

Your back muscles can be developed and thickened by including rowing-type exercises in the programme. Using a closer grip for pulldown-type exercises will also help develop thickness.

Symmetry programme for a flat upper back

Exercise	Sets	Reps
Lat pulldowns (close grip)	3—4	10—12
One-arm rows	3—4	8—12
Seated cable rows	3—4	10—12

High lats

High or short lats make your upper back look flared, but the taper ends just underneath the shoulder blades rather than continuing down to the waist. This creates a long-waisted appearance. The latissimus dorsi attach a little higher up the back, rather than close to the hips. Obviously the natural attachment point cannot be changed but you can dramatically improve the appearance of your back by fully developing the lats along their entire length. Your programme should include movements which emphasise the lower portion of the lats. Technique is very important: ensure that you achieve a full stretch at the end of each repetition and a full contraction at the mid-point. If you shorten the movement, the lower lats will not receive optimal stimulation.

Symmetry programme for high lats

Exercise	Sets	Reps
Chins (parallel grip)	2—3	8—10 (or as many as possible, if less than 8)
Chins (reverse grip)	2—3	8—10 (or as many as possible, if less than 8)
Lat pulldowns (reverse grip)	3	8—12
Seated cable rows	3	8—12

Weak lower back

The muscles of your lower back, the spinal erectors, are easily over-stretched and weakened through poor posture, bearing uneven and heavy loads, sudden twisting, poor exercise technique or lack of direct exercise. They can be strengthened by specific exercises, but also by practising safe technique during exercises such as the squat and dead lift which place considerable stress on the lower back. By holding the abdominals taut during these exercises, indeed during all exercises, you will help avoid injury and strain to the lower back muscles.

Symmetry programme for a weak lower back

Exercise	Sets	Reps
Hyperextensions	4	12—20
Dead lifts or squats	4	12—15

Shoulders

The muscles

The shoulder muscles are comprised of three distinct portions or heads collectively known as the deltoids, a term derived from the Greek 'delta', owing to their geometrically triangular shape. Each head serves a particular function. The anterior (front) deltoid lifts the arm forwards and upwards; the medial (outer) deltoid lifts the arm away from the mid-line of the body to the side (abduction); and the posterior (rear) deltoid lifts the arm to the rear or draws the elbow backwards behind the shoulders.

Shoulder presses (behind the neck; barbell) (*see* page 162)

Muscles developed: deltoids, triceps.
To a lesser extent: the upper pectorals, trapezius and upper back muscles.

Starting position
- ◆ Sit on an upright bench, angled at 75—90 degrees, so that your lower back is firmly in contact with the bench.
- ◆ Hold the bar with your hands just over shoulder-width apart and facing forwards.
- ◆ Remove the bar from the barbell stand (ideally with the help of a training partner), and rest it across the back of your neck.

The movement
- ◆ Press the bar directly upwards over your head and straighten your arms.
- ◆ Bring the bar slowly back to the starting position.

Tips
◆ Keep your elbows in line with your hands throughout.
◆ Keep your back still and upright – don't lean backwards or arch your back as you press the bar upwards as this will strain your lower back.
◆ Hold your abdominal muscles taut to help stabilise your spine or, if you are using a heavy weight, wear a weightlifting belt.

Variations
Front of neck (military) press   Start with the bar resting across the front of your shoulders and push it directly upwards past your face using a shoulder-width grip. This variation places more emphasis on the anterior deltoids and upper pectorals.

Wide grip press   Placing your hands just over shoulder-width apart puts more stress on the deltoids.

Narrow grip press   Placing your hands shoulder-width apart puts more stress on the triceps.

Dumbbell presses (*see* page 162)

Muscles developed: deltoids, triceps.
To a lesser extent: the upper pectorals, trapezius and upper back muscles.

Starting position
◆ Sit on an upright bench, angled at 75—90 degrees, so that your lower back is firmly in contact with the bench.
◆ Hold a pair of dumbbells, hands facing forwards, level with your shoulders.

The movement
◆ Press the dumbbells directly upwards over your head.
◆ Straighten your arms but don't lock out your elbows.
◆ Lower the dumbbells slowly back to the starting position

Tips
◆ Keep your back still and upright – don't lean backwards or arch your spine as you press the bar upwards as this will strain your lower back.
◆ Hold your abdominal muscles taut to help stabilise your spine or,

if you are using a heavy weight, wear a weightlifting belt.
◆ The dumbbells should almost touch at the top of the movement.
◆ Lower the dumbbells until they touch your shoulders – don't shorten the movement.

Variations
Rotate the dumbbells through 90 degrees as you lift them up so that your hands face each other at the top of the movement.

Lateral raises (*see* page 162)

Muscles developed: medial (outside) head of the deltoids.
To a lesser extent: trapezius, anterior (front) head of the deltoids.

Starting position
◆ Stand with your feet hip-width apart.
◆ Hold a dumbbell in each hand, bend forwards slightly and bring the dumbbells in front of your thighs. Your hands should face each other.

The movement
◆ Raise the dumbbells out to the sides, simultaneously turning your hands so that they face the floor.
◆ Raise them until your elbows and hands are level with your shoulders.
◆ Slowly return to the starting position, resisting the weight on the way back down.

Tips
◆ Your little finger should be higher than your thumb at the top of the movement, as if you were pouring water from a jug.
◆ Do not swing the dumbbells out or lean back as you raise the dumbbells – keep your body still.
◆ Lead with your elbows rather than your hands.
◆ Keep your elbows bent at about 10 degrees throughout to avoid straining them.

Variations
Single arm   Lateral raises can be performed using one arm at a time. Hold onto the back of an upright bench or machine with the other hand to help keep you steady. This allows you to concentrate

fully on the movement and helps to prevent you swinging the dumbbells upwards.

Cable lateral raises   The movement can be performed using a low pulley machine. You will need to use a lighter weight but this keeps more continuous tension on the deltoids.

Upright rows (*see* page 162)

Muscles developed: medial (outside) head of the deltoids, trapezius.
To a lesser extent: biceps, forearms.

Starting position
◆ Stand with your feet shoulder-width apart.
◆ Hold the barbell with your hands about 6 inches apart, palms facing towards your body. The bar should rest against the front of your thighs.

The movement
◆ Pull the bar directly upwards towards your chin, bending your elbows out to the sides, until the bar is level with your neck.
◆ Hold for a moment then slowly lower the bar back to the starting position.

Tips
◆ Keep the bar very close to your body throughout the movement.
◆ Make sure you don't sway backwards as you lift the bar.
◆ At the top of the movement your elbows should be level with, or slightly higher than, your hands.
◆ Lower the bar slowly, resisting the weight.

Variations
Wide grip   Using a slightly wider grip of about 10 inches places more emphasis on the deltoids and less on the trapezius.

Bent-over lateral raises

Muscles developed: posterior (rear) head of the deltoids.
To a lesser extent: trapezius, upper back muscles.

Starting position
- ◆ Sit on the end of a bench with only half of your thighs supported.
- ◆ Place your feet and knees together, bend forwards from the waist and hold a pair of dumbbells underneath your thighs with your palms facing each other.

The movement
- ◆ Raise the dumbbells out to the sides, simultaneously turning your hands so that they face the floor.
- ◆ Raise them until your elbows and hands are level with your shoulders.
- ◆ Slowly return to the starting position, resisting the weight on the way down.

Tips
- ◆ Your little finger should be higher than your thumb at the top of the movement, as if you were pouring water from a jug.
- ◆ At the top of the movement, your head, shoulders, elbows and hands should be in a straight line.
- ◆ Keep your torso steady – do not raise your body as you raise the dumbbells.
- ◆ Lead with your elbows rather than your hands.
- ◆ Keep your elbows bent at about 10 degrees throughout to avoid straining them.

Variations
Standing bent-over laterals (*see* page 162)   The movement can be performed from a standing position. Stand with your feet hip-width apart, bend forwards from the waist and hold the dumbbells directly below the shoulders (arms straight). Do not use a heavy weight or attempt this if you have a weak lower back as it may place more stress on the lower back.

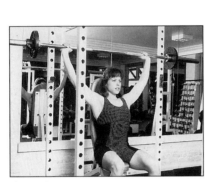

Shoulder presses
(behind the neck; barbell)

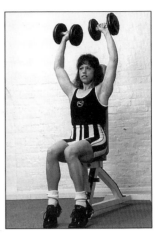

Dumbbell presses

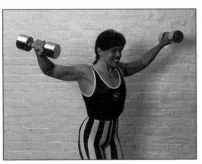

Lateral raises

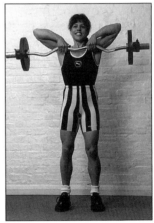

Upright rows

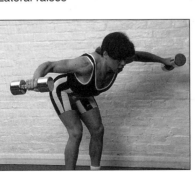

Standing bent-over lateral raises

Symmetry problems

Narrow shoulders

Narrow shoulders greatly affect your total body symmetry. In women, narrow underdeveloped shoulders accentuate a pear shape, making the hips appear wider than they actually are. In men, narrow shoulders make the whole body look weak and undeveloped, or detract from an otherwise athletic physique. Sometimes, the medial (outer) head is poorly developed relative to the anterior (front) head. This is common in weight trainers who focus on chest exercises such as the bench press, at the expense of shoulder exercises.

The width of your shoulders is determined partly by the length of your clavicle (collar) bones and partly by the amount of muscle mass development. Obviously, you cannot change the former but you can significantly increase the width of your shoulders and greatly improve your overall body symmetry by developing your deltoids. The medial (outer) head is mostly responsible for creating width but all three heads need to be developed equally to create good symmetry and avoid injury.

To widen the shoulders, you need to build up the muscle mass by focusing on compound exercises such as shoulder presses and upright rows. These place the greatest stimulus on the shoulders and therefore lead to fastest gains in size and strength. You should also include lateral raises as these directly work the medial head and create width.

Symmetry programme for narrow shoulders

Exercise	Sets	Reps
Shoulder presses (barbell or dumbbell)	3—4	6—10
Upright rows	3—4	6—10
Lateral raises	3—4	6—10

Round or drooping shoulders

Round shoulders are the result of poor posture, bad sitting position, poor muscle strength in the upper back and lack of flexibility in the chest muscles. Viewed from the side, your head juts forwards, your upper back is rounded, your rib cage is reduced or even hollowed and your shoulders droop. It is one of the most common posture faults in men and women.

Round shoulders are also common in weight trainers who have overly developed the anterior head of the shoulders relative to the posterior head. Thus, the anterior head receives disproportionately more stress than the medial and posterior heads, creating muscle imbalance.

The solution is to strengthen the trapezius and muscles of the upper back which will pull the shoulders back into correct alignment; to stretch the chest muscles which will expand the rib cage and allow the shoulders to move back easily into alignment; and to strengthen the shoulder muscles, especially the posterior head, which will correct the muscle imbalance.

Symmetry programme for round shoulders

Exercise	*Sets*	*Reps*
Upright rows	2—3	8—12
Low pulley (cable) rows	2—3	8—12
Shoulder presses (barbell or dumbbell)	2—3	8—12
Bent-over lateral raises	2—3	8—12
Dumbbell flyes	2—3	8—12

17

Chest

The muscles

The largest muscle of the chest is the pectoralis major which attaches to the collar bone (clavicle) and the sternum, and inserts on the upper arm bone (humerus). It flexes the shoulder in a pushing plane of movement, lifting the arm forwards; and in a horizontal plane of movement, bringing the arm from an outstretched position at the side of the body to the centre line of the body (as in the chest flye).

Bench presses (*see* page 169)

Muscles developed: pectorals.
To a lesser extent: deltoids (anterior head) and triceps.

Starting position
- ◆ Lie on your back on a flat bench, ideally with an attached barbell rack. If you have an excessive arch in your back, place your feet on the end of the bench.
- ◆ Hold the bar with your hands just over shoulder-width apart, palms facing forwards.
- ◆ Remove the bar from the barbell rack and position it directly over your chest with your arms fully extended.

The movement
- ◆ Bend your arms, allowing your elbows to travel out to the sides, and slowly lower the bar down to your chest. The bar should touch your upper chest just above your nipple line.
- ◆ Push the bar back to the starting position.

Tips
- ◆ Do not arch your back as you push the bar upwards.
- ◆ Do not bounce the bar off your chest or use the momentum of the weight to complete the repetition.
- ◆ Keep your palms facing forwards and your wrists straight.

Variations
Wide grip Using a grip of one-and-a-half-times shoulder-width places more emphasis on the pectorals (especially the outer part) and less on the triceps.

Narrow grip Using a shoulder-width grip places more emphasis on the triceps and the inner pectorals.

Machine The press may be performed on a Smith machine or a chest press machine.

Dumbbell chest presses (*see* page 169)

Muscles developed: pectorals.
To a lesser extent: deltoids (anterior head) and triceps.

Starting position
- ◆ Lie on your back on a flat or incline bench. If you have an excessive arch in your back, place your feet on the end of the bench.
- ◆ Hold a pair of dumbbells with your palms facing forwards and your arms fully extended, positioned directly over your chest.

The movement
- ◆ Slowly lower the dumbbells down to your armpit area.
- ◆ Hold the position for a moment then press the dumbbells back to the starting position.

Tips
- ◆ Do not arch your back as you push the dumbbells upwards.
- ◆ Lower the dumbbells as far as you can, aiming for a maximum stretch.
- ◆ Do not shorten the downwards movement.
- ◆ Do not lock your arms out fully at the top of the movement.

Incline bench presses (*see* page 169)

Muscles developed: upper pectorals.
To a lesser extent: deltoids (anterior head) and triceps.

Starting position
- Lie on an incline bench, angled at between 30 and 60 degrees (the steeper the incline, the greater the stress on the upper pectorals and anterior deltoids). Ideally the bench should have an attached barbell rack.
- Hold the bar with your hands shoulder-width apart, palms facing forwards. Remove the bar from the barbell rack so it is positioned directly over your collar bone with your arms fully extended.

The movement
- Bend your arms, allowing your elbows to travel out to the sides, and slowly lower the bar down to your chest.
- The bar should just touch the upper part of your chest beneath your collar bone.
- Push the bar back to the starting position.

Tips
- Do not arch your back as you push the bar upwards.
- Do not bounce the bar off your chest or use the momentum of the weight to complete the repetition.
- Keep your palms facing forwards and your wrists straight.

Variations

Dumbbell incline press   The movement may be performed using a pair of dumbbells instead of the barbell. Lower the dumbbells to your armpit area until they just touch your shoulders.

Decline press   The movement may be performed on a specially designed decline bench, angled at approximately 30 degrees, using either a barbell or a pair of dumbbells. This increases the involvement of the lower pectorals.

Dumbbell flyes (*see* page 169)

Muscles developed: pectorals.
To a lesser extent: deltoids (anterior head).

Starting position

◆ Lie on your back on a flat bench. If you have an excessive arch in your back, place your feet on the end of the bench.

◆ Hold a dumbbell in each hand, and hold them above your chest with your arms extended and palms facing each other.

The movement

◆ Slowly lower the dumbbells outwards and downwards in a semi-circular arc until they are level with your shoulders.

◆ As you breathe out, return the dumbbells to the starting position following the same arc.

Tips

◆ Contract your pectorals hard as you bring the dumbbells back to the starting position. Hold for a moment before commencing the next repetition.

◆ Keep a very slight bend (10—15 degrees) in your elbows throughout the movement. Do not bend them more than 15 degrees as you lower the dumbbells out to the sides otherwise you will reduce the stress on the pectorals and increase the involvement of the triceps so the movement becomes more like a press.

◆ Move your arms in a smooth arc.

Variations

Incline flyes Performing flyes on an incline bench set at 30—45 degrees increases the stress placed on the upper pectorals. It is therefore particularly good for developing mass and thickness in the upper chest.

Decline flyes Performing flyes on a decline bench angled at approximately 30 degrees increases the stress placed on the lower pectorals.

Pec dec flyes (*see* page 169)

Muscles developed: pectorals.
To a lesser extent: deltoids (anterior head).

Starting position

◆ Sit on the seat of the pec dec machine, ensuring your lower back is pressed against the back support and adjusting the seat height

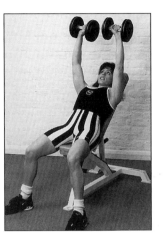

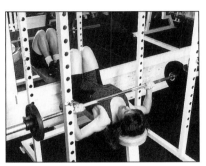

Bench presses

Dumbbell chest presses

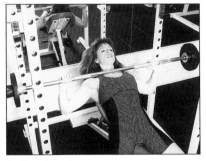

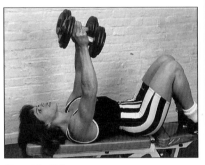

Incline bench presses

Dumbbell flyes

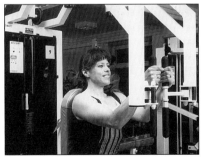

Pec dec flyes

so that your elbows and shoulders are level with the bottom of the pads.

♦ Place your forearms against the pads. Check that your shoulders and elbows make a horizontal line.

The movement

♦ Move the pads towards each other until they just touch in front of your chest.
♦ Hold for a count of two then slowly return the pads to the starting position.

Tips

♦ Contract your pectorals hard at the mid-point.
♦ Do not curl your shoulders forwards as you bring the pads together.
♦ Do not jerk the pads together.
♦ Return the pads slowly, resisting the weight as much as possible.

Cable crossovers

Muscles developed: pectorals.
To a lesser extent: deltoids (anterior head).

Starting position

♦ Attach handles to two overhead pulley machines.
♦ Hold the handles, palms facing down, and stand mid-way between the machines with your feet hip-width apart. Your arms should be fully extended so you achieve a good stretch on your pectorals.
♦ Bend forwards slightly from the waist and maintain this position throughout the exercise.

The movement

♦ Draw the handles towards each other in front of your body, aiming for a point approximately 12 inches in front of your hips.
♦ Allow the handles to cross over by 1—2 inches and hold for a count of two.
♦ Slowly return the handles to the starting position.

Tips

♦ Squeeze your pectorals hard at the mid-point.

- Keep your chest out throughout the movement – do not curl your shoulders forwards as you bring the handles together.
- Move the handles in a slow smooth arc – do not jerk them together.
- Keep your arms slightly bent at an angle of 10—15 degrees throughout.

Dumbbell pullovers

Muscles developed: pectorals, latissimus dorsi (mid-back), serratus, intercostals.

Starting position
- Lie across a flat bench with only your shoulders and upper back supported and your feet flat on the floor, shoulder-width apart.
- Hold a dumbbell with both hands, turned so that your palms are against the inside of one end plate. Hold the dumbbell above your chest with your arms extended.

The movement
- Slowly lower the dumbbell behind your head, keeping your arms almost straight, until your elbows are level with your ears and your hands are just beyond the top of your head.
- Allow your hips to drop down as you lower the dumbbell.
- Pull the dumbbell slowly back to the starting position.

Tips
- Do not allow your hips to rise up as you lower the dumbbell.
- Inhale deeply as you lower the dumbbell and exhale as you return it to the starting position.
- Keep a slight bend in your elbows (10—15 degrees).

Symmetry problems

Flat/narrow chest

A narrow chest has a straight appearance and makes the shoulders appear rounded and dominating. Viewed from the side your chest appears flat or even hollow.

The width and circumference of your chest depends partly on your bone structure, in particular the size and shape of your rib cage and your clavicles (collar bones), and the size of your pectoral muscles. Thus a narrow chest can be improved by building up the pectorals and stretching the muscles between the ribs (serratus and intercostals). Poor posture can also exacerbate the symmetry problem, making the chest appear concave. Thus a two-fold strategy is needed to correct the posture fault (*see* chapter 3) and develop the pectorals and surrounding muscles. This programme is designed to build the pectoral muscles and expand the rib cage by stretching and developing the serratus and intercostals.

Symmetry programme for a narrow chest

Exercise	Sets	Reps
Bench presses (wide grip)	2—3	8—12
Dumbbell presses (alternate with incline d/b presses)	2—3	8—12
Flyes	2—3	8—12
Dumbbell pullovers	2—3	8—12

Concave upper chest

Viewed from the side, the upper part of your chest appears flat or concave and lacks a pleasing aesthetic curve from the collar bone. This symmetry problem is very common, particularly in women who have dieted, since the upper pectorals easily atrophy when calorie and protein intake is reduced over a period of time. A concave upper chest is due to underdevelopment of the upper portion of the pectorals, and so building these up corrects this problem and creates a fuller, more symmetrical chest. It also adds cleavage!

Symmetry programme for a concave upper chest

Exercise	Sets	Reps
Incline bench presses	3—4	8—12
Incline dumbbell presses	3—4	8—12
Incline flyes	3—4	8—12

Flat inner chest

The inner part of your chest appears flat and there is no obvious cleavage line. In women, the breasts appear further apart; in men, the sternum region is flat, making the whole chest region look shallow. The problem may be due to a naturally wide rib cage or to underdevelopment of the inner part of the pectorals. The solution is therefore to select exercises which stress the inner pectorals, as this will re-balance the chest muscles and create a more symmetrical cleavage.

Symmetry programme for a flat inner chest

Exercise	Sets	Reps
Bench presses (narrow grip)	2—3	8—12
Pec dec flyes	2—3	8—12
Cable crossovers	2—3	8—12

18

Abdominals

The muscles

The abdominals are comprised of four main muscle groups: the internal and external obliques, running diagonally from the lower ribs to opposite hip, which twist the trunk; the rectus abdominis, running from your pubic bone to your lower ribs, which flexes the spine; and the transverse abdominis, a flat sheath of muscle running across the torso which acts as a muscular girdle to support the contents of the abdomen.

◆ *Technique note* ◆

The key to safe and effective abdominal exercising is technique. You should concentrate on each part of the movement, keeping it slow and controlled. Don't worry about how far you are moving – it's the feel that is most important. Concentrate on each movement, feeling the contraction through the full range. When it starts to hurt (not to be confused with actual pain), take a short rest then complete the exercise or move onto the next.

Curl ups (*see* page 177)

Muscles developed: rectus abdominis (upper part).

Starting position
◆ Lie on your back, knees bent and feet on the floor hip-width apart.

◆ There should be a small gap, approximately two fingers' depth, between your lower back and the floor.
◆ Place your hands on your thighs.

The movement
◆ Breathe in. As you breathe out, pull your abdomen in and slowly round your spine forwards to lift your head, shoulders and upper back off the floor, at the same time sliding your hands down your thighs to your knees. Keep your abdomen flat.
◆ Hold for a count of two.
◆ Slowly return to the start position.

Tips
◆ Your lower and middle back should remain on the floor.
◆ Lift only as far as you are able while holding your abdomen flat.
◆ Make sure you use your abdominals. Lead with the chest – don't let your head or neck initiate the movement.

Variations
Changing the position of your arm makes this exercise more of a challenge. Place your fingers at the sides of your head, elbows out, so that you can support the weight of your head. Make sure you do not pull your head up with your hands, though; use your abdominals.

One-leg-up abdominal curls (*see* page 177)

Muscles developed: rectus abdominis.

Starting position
◆ Lie on your back, one leg bent with the foot on the floor.
◆ Raise the other leg straight so your knees are side by side.
◆ Place your hands by the sides of your head.

The movement
◆ As you breathe out, curl your head, shoulders and upper back up and try to extend your straight leg even further.
◆ Slowly return to the start position.
◆ After the required number of repetitions, repeat using the other leg.

Tips
- ◆ Keep your elbows back and relaxed.
- ◆ Hold at the top of the movement for a second or two before uncurling.

The crunch (*see* page 177)

Muscles developed: rectus abdominis.

Starting position
- ◆ Lie on the floor, with your knees bent and ankles crossed above your hips. Place your hands by the sides of your head, elbows out.

The movement
- ◆ As you breathe out, curl your head, shoulders and upper back towards your knees.
- ◆ Hold in the contracted position for a count of two.
- ◆ Let your body uncurl slowly back to the starting position.

Tips
- ◆ Your lower back should remain firmly on the floor. If you rise any higher than 45 degrees you shift the emphasis from your abdominals to your hip flexors which can strain the lower back.
- ◆ Focus on moving your ribs towards your hips.
- ◆ Do not pull your head with your hands – keep your elbows out and relaxed.

Variations
For a more advanced exercise, extend your arms above your head – this increases the leverage.

Reverse crunches (*see* page 177)

Muscles developed: rectus abdominis (lower part).

Starting position
- ◆ Lie on the floor with your knees bent over your hips and your ankles crossed (the same position as for crunches).
- ◆ Place your arms on the floor alongside your body, palms flat on the floor. Press your lower back to the floor.

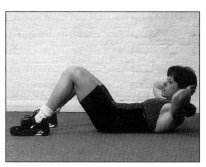

Curl up (variation: fingers at the sides of the head)

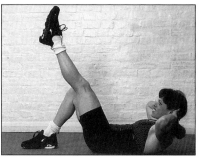

One-leg-up abdominal curls

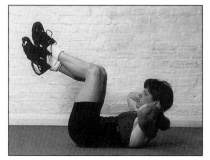

The crunch

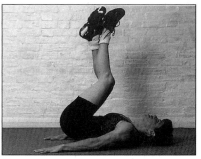

Reverse crunches

The movement
◆ Curl your hips 1—2 inches off the floor, aiming your knees towards your chest. Press your arms down to help you.
◆ Hold for a count of two.
◆ Slowly return to the starting position.

Tips
◆ This should be a controlled, deliberate movement. Do not jerk or bounce your hips off the floor; curl one vertebra up at a time.
◆ As you start the movement, contract your abdominals.
◆ Do not allow your abdominals to relax at the top of the movement or whilst you are uncurling.
◆ Uncurl slowly – do not allow your hips to simply fall back to the floor.

Oblique crunches (*see* page 180)

Muscles developed: internal and external obliques.

Starting position
◆ Lie on your back with your right leg bent and the foot flat on the floor.
◆ Place your left foot across your right knee.
◆ Place your hands by the sides of your head, elbows pointing outwards.

The movement
◆ As you breathe out, lift your right shoulder and aim it towards your left knee.
◆ Hold for one or two seconds, then return to your starting position as you breathe in.
◆ Repeat using alternate legs.

Tips
◆ Imagine your rib cage rotating to the side as you curl up.
◆ Lead with your shoulder rather than your elbow.
◆ Make sure you lower your body slowly back to the floor.
◆ Do not twist your head, only your torso.

Lying side bends (*see* page 180)

Muscles developed: obliques.

Starting position
◆ Lie on your side with your knees slightly bent.
◆ Place your top arm behind your head.

The movement
◆ As you breathe out, raise your head and shoulders a short distance off the floor, aiming your ribs towards your top hip.
◆ Hold for a second then breathe in as you return to the starting position.
◆ Repeat to the other side.

Tips
◆ Imagine you are reducing the space between your ribs and hips.
◆ Don't worry if you don't reach up very far – concentrate on feeling the movement.
◆ Keep your head in line with your body – don't jerk it upwards.

The flattener (*see* page 180)

Muscles developed: transverse abdominis.

Starting position
◆ Stand sideways in front of a mirror with your feet hip-width apart.

The movement
◆ Focus on the muscles of your abdomen. As you breathe out, flatten your muscles without moving your body. Imagine you are tightening a flat sheet across your abdomen.
◆ Breathe in, relaxing your abdominals and repeat.

Tips
◆ This is a very subtle movement requiring concentration and practice. Watch the mirror carefully.
◆ Make sure you don't move your hips or your rib cage.

Variations
The movement may be performed on all fours or in a seated position.

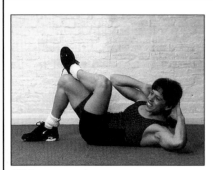

Oblique crunches

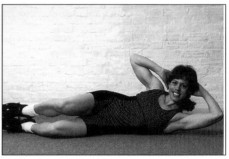

Lying side bends

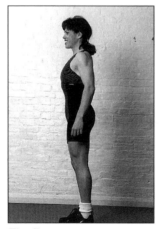

The flattener

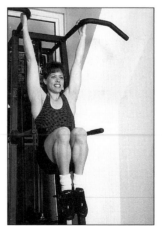

Hanging leg raises

Hanging leg raises (*see* page 180)

Muscles developed: rectus abdominis, hip flexors.

Starting position
◆ Hang from a high bar with your hands shoulder-width apart.
◆ Bend your knees.

The movement
◆ Raise your knees until they are level with your hips, curling your hips towards your rib cage.
◆ Hold for a moment then slowly return your knees to the starting position.

Tips
◆ Your torso should remain in a straight line.
◆ Do not swing your knees up or use the momentum of your legs – use the strength of your abdominals to move your hips and legs.
◆ Do not allow your body to swing – keep it still!

◆ *Back strain?* ◆

Weak abdominals are often associated with back problems. This is because slack abdominal muscles become over-stretched, causing the pelvis to tilt forwards creating an excessive arch in the lower back and potential back pain.

Strong abdominals support and stabilise the pelvis and lower back. Strengthening these muscles (and stretching the hip flexors) will eliminate excessive arching in the lower back, give good posture and minimise potential back problems.

Symmetry problems

Lower tummy bulge

Viewed from the side, the lower part of your tummy appears rounded and protruding. This is due to poor posture, poor muscle tone in the lower abdominals, overstretched abdominals and, possibly, an accumulation of fat. The posture problem, *lordosis*, is caused by an excessive forwards pelvic tilt. The hip flexors (which connect the thigh bone with the lower vertebrae) become tighter and pull and compress the lower vertebrae, leading to excessive arching in your lower back.

The solution is to correct the pelvic tilt, stretch the hip flexors and strengthen the abdominals (especially the lower region). Body fat should be reduced if necessary by increasing aerobic activity (aim for 3—5 sessions per week of 20—45 minutes), and cutting calories by 250—500 kcal per day. Cut down on high fat foods such as fatty meats, spreading fats, chips, crisps, chocolates, pastries, cakes and biscuits, and replace high fat snacks with fresh fruit, dried fruit, low calorie yoghurt and toast/bread.

Symmetry programme for a lower tummy bulge

Exercise	Sets	Reps
The crunch	1—2	20—25
Reverse crunches	1—2	20—25
Hanging leg raises (only when advanced)	1—2	15—20
The flattener	1—2	15—20
Hip flexor stretches (page 118)		Minimum 15 seconds

Wide waist

Viewed from the side your waist appears wide relative to the hips and chest and your tummy may protrude slightly. This is usually due to an excess of fat stored at the sides of the waist, poor muscle tone of the obliques and a 'short' waist structure.

As I have explained, fat stored at the sides of the waist cannot be spot reduced by diet or exercise. However, it can be reduced when overall body fat levels are reduced through increasing aerobic activity (3—5 sessions per week of 20—45 minutes) and cutting calories by 250—500 kcal per day. Again, cut down on high fat foods such as fatty meats, spreading fats, chips, crisps, chocolates, pastries, cakes and biscuits, and replace high fat snacks with fresh fruit, dried fruit, low calorie yoghurt and toast/bread.

You can dramatically improve your appearance by strengthening the oblique muscles. This will create a narrower waistline and better posture. Unfortunately, your basic skeletal structure cannot be changed. A naturally short mid-section is determined by the distance between your ribs and pelvis and can make the waist appear wider than it actually is. However, you can still improve your appearance by toning the abdominal muscles, particularly the obliques.

Symmetry programme for a wide waist

Exercise	Sets	Reps
Oblique crunches	1—2	20—25
Lying side bends	1—2	20—25
Curl ups or crunches	1—2	15—20
Reverse crunches	1—2	15—20

Arms

The muscles

Approximately 60% of the upper arm muscle mass is comprised of the triceps; 30% is comprised of the biceps; and the other 10% comes from the brachialis muscles lying beneath the biceps.

The biceps muscles have three functions: to flex (bend) the arm; to supinate or twist the forearm; and to assist in raising the shoulder forwards.

The triceps muscle has three distinct heads – the long inner head, the medial head and the shorter, outer (lateral) head that gives the familiar horseshoe appearance to the outside upper arm. The collective function of the heads of the triceps is to partially or fully straighten the arm from a bent position. While it is difficult to isolate each triceps head, different exercises place greater emphasis on individual heads.

Barbell curls (*see* page 190)

Muscles developed: biceps.
To a lesser extent: forearms.

Starting position
◆ Stand with your feet hip-width apart.
◆ Hold a barbell with your hands shoulder-width apart, palms facing forwards.
◆ The bar should rest against your thighs and your arms should be fully extended.

The movement
- ◆ Bend your arms as you curl the bar up in a smooth arc towards your shoulders. Keep your upper arms fixed by the sides of your body.
- ◆ Pause for a count of two then slowly lower the bar back to the starting position.

Tips
- ◆ Do not move your upper arms at any point of the movement.
- ◆ Keep your body absolutely still – make sure you don't lean back or swing the bar up as this will strain the back and reduce the work on the biceps.
- ◆ Keep your wrists locked.
- ◆ Lower the bar very slowly (take at least 3—4 seconds) until your arms are fully extended – shortening or rushing the downwards phase will reduce the effectiveness of the exercise.

Variations
EZ bar curls   Arm curls can be performed using an EZ bar instead of a straight bar. This reduces the stress on the wrists although it puts the biceps in a biometrically weaker position.

Wide grip curls   Using a grip slightly greater than shoulder-width places more emphasis on the inner head of the biceps.

Narrow grip curls   Using a grip slightly narrower than shoulder-width places more emphasis on the outer head of the biceps.

Preacher curls

Muscles developed: biceps (particularly lower portion).
To a lesser extent: forearms.

Starting position
- ◆ Sit on the seat of a preacher curl machine, adjusting it so that your armpits rest over the top edge of the pad.
- ◆ Hold a barbell with your hands shoulder-width apart, palms facing forwards.
- ◆ Your arms should be fully extended.

The movement
- ◆ Bend your arms as you curl the bar up in a smooth arc towards your shoulders, stopping about 9—12 inches short of your shoulders.

185

◆ Pause for a count of two then slowly lower the bar back to the starting position.

Tips
◆ Keep your shoulders back and relaxed – avoid leaning forwards as you curl the bar up.
◆ Keep your body still and your wrists locked.
◆ Lower the bar until your arms are fully extended – shortening the downwards phase will reduce the effectiveness of the exercise.

Variations
EZ bar preacher curls   Preacher curls can be performed using an EZ bar instead of a straight bar. This reduces the stress on the wrists although it puts the biceps in a biometrically weaker position.

Wide grip EZ preacher curls   Using a grip slightly greater than shoulder-width places more emphasis on the outer head of the biceps.

Narrow grip EZ preacher curls   Using a grip slightly narrower than shoulder-width places more emphasis on the inner head of the biceps.

Dumbbell preacher curls   Preacher curls can be performed with dumbbells. Perform them one arm at a time, allowing you to concentrate fully on each rep.

Dumbbell curls (*see* page 190)

Muscles developed: biceps.
To a lesser extent: forearms.

Starting position
◆ Stand with your feet hip-width apart or sit at the end of a bench.
◆ Hold a pair of dumbbells, palms facing inwards towards your body.
◆ Your arms should be fully extended.

The movement
◆ Curl one dumbbell up at a time in a smooth arc towards your shoulders, smoothly rotating your forearm so that your palm faces your shoulder at the top of the movement.

- Pause for a count of two then slowly lower the dumbbell back to the starting position.
- Repeat using alternate arms.

Tips
- Curl the dumbbells up slowly – do not swing them up.
- Keep your upper arms fixed by the sides of your body.
- Keep your body absolutely still – make sure you don't sway back.
- Keep your wrists locked.
- Make sure you fully straighten your arms when you lower the dumbbells; do not shorten the downwards phase.

Variations
Incline curls   Performing dumbbells on an incline bench set at 45 degrees works the lower portion of the biceps. Again, make sure you start and finish the movement with straight arms.

Concentration curls (*see* page 190)

Muscles developed: biceps.
To a lesser extent: forearms.

Starting position
- Sit on a bench with your legs wide apart. Hold a dumbbell with one hand and brace that arm against the inside of the same thigh. Your arm should be straight and your palm should be facing the opposite thigh.

The movement
- Slowly curl the dumbbell up in a smooth arc towards your shoulder.
- Pause for a count of two then slowly lower the dumbbell back to the starting position.
- Repeat using alternate legs.

Tips
- Make sure you curl the dumbbell to your shoulder and don't move your shoulder to the dumbbell. Keep your shoulder back and relaxed.
- Do not lean backwards.

- Keep your upper arm fixed.
- Make sure you fully straighten your arms when you lower the dumbbells; do not shorten the downwards phase.

Lying cable curls

Muscles developed: biceps.
To a lesser extent: forearms.

Starting position
- Attach a short bar to the overhead cable of a lat machine.
- Place a bench in front of the machine and lie down on your back facing away from the machine.
- Grasp the bar with your hands shoulder-width apart and facing the machine.
- Your arms should be fully extended and perpendicular to your body, by your ears.

The movement
- Keeping your upper arms still, bend your elbows and curl the bar until it is beyond the top of your head.
- Pause for a count of two then slowly return the bar to the starting position.

Tips
- Keep your elbows stationary.
- Do not allow your hips to rise from the bench.
- Keep your wrists locked throughout.
- Make sure you fully straighten your arms after completing each rep.

Triceps pushdowns (*see* page 190)

Muscles developed: triceps (especially the outer head).
To a lesser extent: forearms.

Starting position
- Attach a short, angled bar to the overhead cable of a lat machine.
- Place your hands on the bar about 6 inches apart, palms facing down.
- Bring the bar down until your elbows are at your sides and bent at about 90 degrees.

The movement

◆ Press the bar down, moving only your forearms, until your arms are straight.
◆ Pause for a count of two then slowly return the bar to the starting position.

Tips

◆ Keep your elbows fixed firmly at your sides throughout the movement.
◆ Do not lean too far forwards.
◆ Keep your wrists locked and your palms facing you.

Variation

You may use a short straight bar instead of the angled bar although this places more strain on the wrists and forearms.

Bench dips (*see* page 190)

Muscles developed: triceps (especially the inner head).

Starting position

◆ Position two benches about the length of your legs apart.
◆ Place your hands shoulder-width apart, fingers facing forwards, on the edge of one bench.
◆ Place your heels on the other bench so that your legs form a straight bridge between the two benches.

The movement

◆ Bend your elbows and lower your body until your elbows make an angle of 90 degrees.
◆ Pause for a moment then straighten your arms back to the starting position.

Tips

◆ Keep your back close to the bench.
◆ Do not lock or snap out your elbows at the top of the movement.
◆ Keep your elbows directed backwards.
◆ Do not shorten the downwards phase.
◆ Keep the movement slow – do not rush the reps.

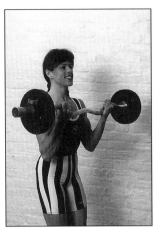

Barbell curls

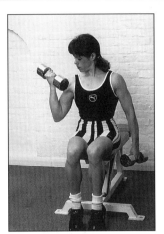

Dumbbell curls

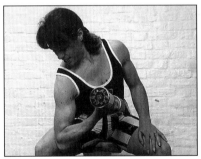

Concentration curls

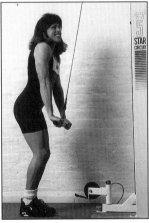

Triceps pushdowns

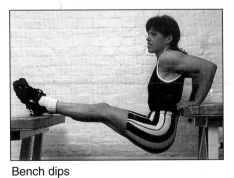

Bench dips

Variations

To make the movement easier, place your feet flat on the floor instead of on a bench. For a more advanced movement, place a weight disc across your lap to increase the resistance.

Dips (*see* page 195)

Muscles developed: triceps (especially the inner head).
To a lesser extent: pectorals.

Starting position
♦ Place your hands on the parallel dipping bars.
♦ Jump up and straighten your arms.
♦ Cross your ankles behind you.

The movement
♦ Bend your arms, keeping your elbows close to your sides, and slowly lower yourself down until your elbows make an angle of 90 degrees.
♦ Pause for a moment then slowly straighten your arms, raising yourself back to the starting position.

Tips
♦ Do not lean forwards – keep as upright as possible.
♦ Keep your elbows in.
♦ Do not shorten the downwards phase of the movement.
♦ Do not lock out or snap out your elbows as you push back up – straighten your arms only about ¾ of the full extension.

Variations

For a more advanced movement, attach a weight belt around your waist to increase the resistance.

Lying triceps extensions (*see* page 195)

Muscles developed: triceps (especially the long inner head and medial head).

Starting position
♦ Lie on your back on a flat bench. If you have an excessive arch in your back, place your feet on the end of the bench.

191

♦ Hold the bar with your hands slightly less than shoulder-width apart, palms facing forwards.

♦ The bar should be positioned directly over your chest with your arms fully extended.

The movement

♦ Keeping your upper arms stationary, bend your elbows as you lower the bar until it is just beyond your head.

♦ Pause for a moment then straighten your arms back to the starting position.

Tips

♦ For maximum muscle development, straighten your arms fully at the end of the movement.

♦ Keep your elbows perfectly still – do not allow them to move out to the sides, or backwards with the bar.

♦ Keep your hips firmly down on the bench.

♦ Lower the bar as far back as you safely can to achieve the greatest range of movement.

Variations

EZ bar The movement may be performed with either a straight bar or an EZ bar.

Lying dumbbell triceps extensions Use a dumbbell instead of a barbell, placing your hands against the inner side of one of the end plates. You may also perform this exercise holding a pair of dumb-bells, palms facing each other.

Lying single-arm triceps extensions Perform the movement using a dumbbell (as above), one arm at a time, palm facing inwards. You may use your free hand to steady your other elbow.

Lying machine triceps extensions Position a bench in front of a low pulley cable machine. Attach a short straight bar to the lower pulley and proceed as for barbell triceps extensions.

Standing triceps extensions The movement may be performed using either a barbell, EZ bar or dumbbell in a standing position. Start with the bar or dumbbell directly above your head and lower it behind your head, bending your elbows to 90 degrees. Make sure you do not arch your back.

Seated triceps extensions The movement may be performed using either a barbell, EZ bar or dumbbell in a seated position on the end of a bench or on a bench angled at 90 degrees to provide back support. Start with the bar or dumbbell directly above your head and lower it behind your head, bending your elbows to 90 degrees. Make sure you do not arch your back.

Cross body triceps extensions

Muscles developed: triceps (especially the outer head).

Starting position
◆ Lie on your back on a flat bench, holding a dumbbell in one hand straight overhead.
◆ Turn your hand so that your thumb points down and your palm faces your legs.

The movement
◆ Keeping your upper arm stationary, bend your elbow and lower the dumbbell across your body towards the opposite shoulder.
◆ Pause for a count of two then straighten your arm back to the starting position.
◆ Repeat using alternate arms.

Tips
◆ Keep your upper arm fixed.
◆ Fully extend your arm at the end of each repetition, squeezing the triceps.
◆ Lower the dumbbell as close to your shoulder as you can – do not shorten the range of movement.

Triceps kickbacks (*see* page 195)

Muscles developed: triceps (especially the outer head).

Starting position
◆ Hold a dumbbell in one hand.
◆ Bend forwards from the waist until your torso is parallel to the floor.
◆ Place your other hand and knee on a bench to stabilise yourself – your back should be flat and horizontal.

◆ Bend the arm holding the dumbbell 90 degrees at the elbow and bring it up so that your upper arm is parallel to and close to the side of your body, and the dumbbell is hanging straight down below the elbow.

The movement
◆ Keeping your elbow stationary, extend your arm backwards until your arm is straight and horizontal.
◆ Hold for a count of two then slowly return to the starting position.
◆ Repeat using alternate arms.

Tips
◆ Extend your arm slowly - do not swing the dumbbell back.
◆ Keep your upper arm fixed.
◆ Keep your lower back flat and still.
◆ Use a relatively light weight as the exercise is harder to perform than many people imagine.

Close grip bench presses (*see* page 195)

Muscles developed: triceps (especially the inner head), inner pectorals.

Starting position
◆ Lie on your back on a flat bench, ideally with an attached barbell rack. If you have an excessive arch in your back, place your feet on the end of the bench.
◆ Hold the bar with your hands slightly less than shoulder-width apart, palms facing forwards.
◆ Remove the bar from the rack and position it directly over your chest with your arms fully extended.

The movement
◆ Bend your arms, keeping your elbows as close to your body as possible, and slowly lower the bar down to your chest. The bar should touch your chest just below your nipple line.
◆ Push the bar back to the starting position.

Tips
◆ Do not arch your back as you push the bar upwards.

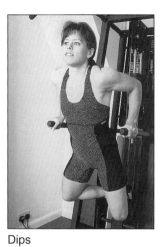

Dips

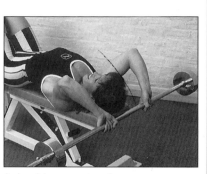

Lying triceps extensions

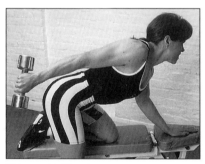

Triceps kickbacks

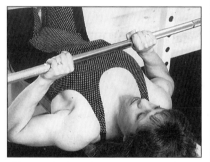

Close grip bench presses

◆ Do not bounce the bar off your chest.
◆ Keep your palms facing forwards and your wrists straight.

Variations
Smith machine   The movement may be performed on a Smith machine.

Symmetry problems

Skinny arms

Poorly-muscled arms are the result of a lack of direct biceps and triceps exercise. Your muscles are small, underdeveloped, lacking in density and appear straight and flat with no discernible shape. The problem can be easily corrected by including mass-building exercises for your arm muscles, such as barbell curls, triceps extensions and triceps pushdowns. These movements recruit the largest number of muscle fibres and therefore place maximum stress on the arm muscles, producing the fastest gains in size and strength.

Your programme should include more triceps work than biceps work because, contrary to popular belief, the triceps muscle is actually responsible for a considerably greater portion of the upper arm muscle mass than the biceps. Many trainers make the mistake of overtraining their biceps and neglecting their triceps in an attempt to get bigger arms.

Symmetry programme for skinny arms

Exercise	Sets	Reps
Barbell curls	2—3	8—12
Incline dumbbell curls	2—3	8—12
Lying triceps extensions	2—3	8—12
Close grip bench presses or dips	2—3	8—12
Triceps pushdowns	2—3	8—12

Bulky shapeless arms

Viewed from the side, your arms appear chunky, straight and lacking in aesthetic appeal and definition. You have developed good muscle mass in the arms but there is no pleasing 'peak' to the biceps nor a pleasing horseshoe outline to the triceps. This problem is partly due to excessive subcutaneous fat covering the muscles' outline and partly to poor exercise technique, shortening the range of movement, leading to sub-optimal development of the muscle along its whole length.

The solution is to gradually reduce body fat, improve your training technique and incorporate more isolation exercises for arms. This will help improve the definition and shape of your biceps and triceps. You need to reduce your overall body fat by cutting your calories by about 250—500 kcal per day (particularly cutting down on fats), and increasing your aerobic activity. Aim to work out for 20—45 minutes, 3—5 times a week.

The programme includes a couple of mass-building exercises – ensure that you achieve the full range of movement and do not shorten the motion – and isolation exercises which place greater demand on different parts of the muscles' length. Use slightly higher reps (up to 15), lower weights and concentrate on the feel of the movement.

Symmetry programme for bulky shapeless arms

Exercise	Sets	Reps
Cable curls	2—3	12—15
Preacher curls (alternated with incline dumbbell curls)	2—3	12—15
Concentration curls	2—3	12—15
One-arm triceps extensions (dumbbell)	2—3	12—15
Triceps kickbacks	2—3	12—15
Dips or bench dips	2—3	12—15

20

Calves

The muscles

The calves are comprised of two muscles: the gastrocnemius and the soleus. The gastrocnemius is the larger of the two and lies on top of the soleus. It is worked when the leg is fully straight, and has two distinct lobes which are visible from behind when the calf is flexed. The soleus is a broad, flat muscle which is located beneath the gastrocnemius. It sweeps out to the sides and over across the shins, and is worked when the knee is bent at about 90 degrees.

Calf raises (*see* page 199)

Muscles developed: gastrocnemius.

Starting position
- Place your shoulders under the pads of a standing calf raise machine.
- Step onto the block and allow your heels to hang off the edge.
- Stand with your feet hip-width apart and pointing directly ahead.
- Straighten your legs as you lift the selected weight clear of the rest of the stack.

The movement
- Rise up on your toes as high as possible.
- Hold the fully contracted position for a count of two then slowly lower your heels down as far as they will go.

Tips
- Keep your legs straight throughout the movement.

- Stretch your calves fully at the bottom of the movement – your heels should be lower than your toes.
- Do not bounce up from the bottom – keep the movement smooth and continuous.

Variations

Toes pointing out   Angling your feet outwards at 45 degrees places more emphasis on the inner part of the calves.

Toes pointing in   Angling your feet inwards at 45 degrees places more emphasis on the outer part of the calves.

Barbell calf raise   Place a barbell across the back of your shoulders and perform the calf raise as above. Place your toes on a low platform or block to increase the range of movement.

Smith machine calf raise   Place your shoulders under the bar of a Smith machine and step onto a low platform or block with your heels hanging off the edge. Perform the calf raise as above.

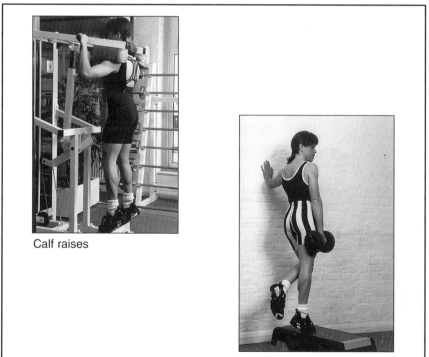

Calf raises

Dumbbell calf raises

Dumbbell calf raises (*see* page 199)

Muscles developed: gastrocnemius.

Starting position
◆ Hold a dumbbell in one hand.
◆ Place the ball of one foot (same side as the hand holding the dumbbell) on the edge of a block or platform, allowing your heel to hang off the edge.
◆ Cross the other foot behind your lower leg.
◆ Hold onto a suitable support with the other hand to steady yourself.

The movement
◆ Rise up on your toes as high as possible.
◆ Hold the fully contracted position for a count of two then slowly lower your heel down as far as it will go.
◆ Repeat using alternate arms and legs.

Tips
◆ Keep your leg straight throughout the movement.
◆ Keep your body upright and allow the dumbbell to hang from your straight arm.
◆ Stretch your calf fully at the bottom of the movement – your heel should be lower than your toes.
◆ Keep the movement smooth and continuous.

Variations
Toes pointing out Angling your feet outwards at 45 degrees places more emphasis on the inner part of the calves.

Toes pointing in Angling your feet inwards at 45 degrees places more emphasis on the outer part of the calves.

Seated calf raises

Muscles developed: soleus.

Starting position
◆ Sit down on a seated calf raise machine, adjusting the height of the pads to the length of your lower legs.
◆ Position your knees under the pads and place your toes on the edge

of the platform. Rise up on your toes just a short way to release the safety catch then lower your heels down as far as possible.

The movement
- ◆ Rise up on your toes as high as possible.
- ◆ Hold the fully contracted position for a count of two then slowly lower your heels down as far as they will go.

Tips
- ◆ Do not hurry the reps or bounce up from the bottom.
- ◆ Stretch your calves fully at the bottom of the movement – your heels should be lower than your toes.

Variations
Toes pointing out   Angling your feet outwards at 45 degrees places more emphasis on the inner part of the calves.

Toes pointing in   Angling your feet inwards at 45 degrees places more emphasis on the outer part of the calves.

Calf presses

Muscles developed: gastrocnemius.

Starting position
- ◆ Sit into the base of a leg press machine.
- ◆ Place the balls of your feet on the bottom of the platform with your heels hanging off the edge. Your legs should be straight and your feet hip-width apart. Release the safety catch.

The movement
- ◆ Press the platform up as high as possible.
- ◆ Hold the fully contracted position for a count of two then slowly lower your heels down as far as they will go.

Tips
- ◆ Keep your legs straight throughout the movement.
- ◆ Stretch your calves fully at the bottom of the movement – your heels should be lower than your toes.
- ◆ Do not bounce up from the bottom – keep the movement smooth and continuous.

Variations

Toes pointing out Angling your feet outwards at 45 degrees places more emphasis on the inner part of the calves.

Toes pointing in Angling your feet inwards at 45 degrees places more emphasis on the outer part of the calves.

Symmetry problems

Small calves

The calves appear thin and straight when viewed from the front, side or back. This may be due partly to genetics and partly to lack of direct calf work. Some people have naturally thin calf muscles owing to a high percentage distribution of slow twitch fibres. These are better suited to endurance work and hypertrophy or increase in size less readily. However, you can still improve the size of your calves through heavy resistance training, which will stimulate the fast twitch (explosive) fibres.

It is a common mistake to neglect calf training. Many trainers leave them until the end of a workout, performing merely one or two sets or omitting them altogether. It is tempting to believe that calves receive sufficient stimulation from everyday activities such as standing and walking, or from jogging or playing other sports, so they do not need to be trained in the gym. However, for most people, the slow twitch fibres in the calves readily adapt to this everyday high volume, low intensity training without increasing in size. To increase their size further your training programme must include high-intensity work.

Symmetry programme for small calves

Exercise	Sets	Reps
Standing calf raises	3—4	12—20
Calf presses	3—4	12—20
Seated calf raises	3—4	12—20

Bulky calves

Big bulky calves may be the envy of those with skinny calves, but here the problem is a lack of shape and symmetry. The circumference of the lower leg barely changes from the knee to the ankle; the calf muscles are large but they are not aesthetically pleasing. Bulky calves are often the consequence of genetic endowment such as a large percentage of fast twitch fibres, or are the result of playing sports such as football, rugby, and other activities involving sprinting during childhood and adolescence. Those born with a high percentage of fast twitch fibres find that their calves readily respond to high-intensity exercise such as sprinting and jumping.

The only way to reduce the size of a muscle is to stop training and allow it to atrophy or waste away. However, this will not improve the shape and symmetry of the muscle – you will end up with a smaller, flabbier version of the original. The solution for bulky calves is to define and shape the muscles. By incorporating movements during which the toes are angled outwards or inwards you will fully stimulate all areas of the calf muscles and so create a pleasing outer and inner sweep to the lower leg.

Concentrate on exercising the gastrocnemius rather than the soleus as it is this muscle which gives the lower leg its curved shape. Chances are that if you have bulky calves extending down to the ankles, the soleus is well developed so you can omit specific soleus exercises. Ensure you perform all exercises with your legs perfectly straight in order to stress the gastrocnemius fully. Use light or moderate weights that allow you to get a full range of movement.

Symmetry programme for bulky calves

Exercise	Sets	Reps
Calf raises (alternate sets with toes angled in and toes angled out)	2—3	15—20
Dumbbell calf raises (alternate sets with toes angled in and toes angled out)	2—3	15—20
Calf presses (alternate sets with toes angled in and toes angled out)	2—3	15—20

High calves

'High' or 'short' calves are characterised by a lack of muscle bulk in the lower calf; the main bulk of the calf muscle is high up on the lower leg, creating an unbalanced curve. The problem is mainly due to a higher insertion point of the gastrocnemius, that is the muscle flare ends rather abruptly halfway down the lower leg. While training cannot alter the insertion point, the appearance of the lower leg can be balanced by developing the soleus muscle. Therefore, gastrocnemius work should be limited and you should concentrate on soleus exercises.

Symmetry programme for high calves

Exercise	Sets	Reps
Seated calf raises (toes straight ahead)	2—3	12—20
Seated calf raises (toes angled out)	2—3	12—20
Seated calf raises (toes angled in)	2—3	12—20

Eating plans

The eating plans below have been designed as a basis for developing your personal daily diet. Each plan provides about 60% energy from carbohydrate, 15—20% from protein and 20—25% from fat. Alternatively, you can plan your daily diet using the suggested serving sizes from each food group.

Estimating your calorie needs

To maintain your weight

Multiply your current weight in pounds by:

15 if you exercise less than 3 times per week
18 if you exercise 3—5 times per week
23 if you exercise more than 5 times per week
28 if you exercise intensely for more than 2 hours per day, 5 times per week

To lose weight

Estimate the number of calories needed to maintain your weight and subtract 500. This will enable you to lose an average of 1 lb per week. Increasing your aerobic activity will produce a faster loss of approximately 2 lbs per week.

To gain weight

Estimate the number of calories needed to maintain your weight and add 500 kcal.

Guide to food portion sizes

Each eating plan is based on portions from all of the main food groups. The portion sizes are detailed in the following guide.

◆ *Fruit and vegetables* ◆	
	Size of one portion
Fresh fruit	1 apple/pear/peach/orange/banana 4 oz (100 g) berries (e.g. strawberries, raspberries) 4 oz (100 g) pineapple/grapes 4 apricots/plums 2 kiwi fruit ½ mango
Tinned fruit	½ tin (14 oz/400 g) of pineapple/peaches/apricots (drained)
Fruit juice	1 glass (3 ½ fl oz/100 ml) juice
Vegetables	In general, 4 oz (100 g) vegetables 2 carrots/courgettes 2 florets broccoli 10 brussels sprouts 3 tbsp peas 2—3 tbsp spinach/cabbage/runner beans
Salad	1 large tomato 3-inch piece cucumber 1 bunch watercress 3 sticks celery 1 cos lettuce/½ iceberg lettuce

◆ *Cereals and starchy vegetables* ◆	
	Size of one portion
Bread	1 thick slice of bread 1 small roll/½ bap/½ bagel ½ large pitta/chappati
Cereals/grains	2 heaped tbsp cooked pasta/rice/noodles 1 oz (25 g) uncooked weight pasta/rice/noodles
Starchy veg	1 small (3 oz/75 g) baked or boiled potato 3 new potatoes

	2 tbsp cooked sweet potato/yam/plantain 2 tbsp sweetcorn 1 large parsnip
Breakfast cereals	1 small bowl (1 oz/25 g) breakfast cereal 2 Weetabix 1 'variety pack' box of cereal
Crackers	3 crackers/crispbreads/rice cakes

◆ *Milk and dairy products* ◆

	Size of one portion
Milk	⅓ pint full fat/semi skimmed/skimmed milk 1 large glass (7 fl oz/200 ml)
Cheese	1 matchbox-sized piece (½ oz/15 g) hard cheese (e.g. Cheddar)/soft ripened cheese (e.g. brie) 1 small pot (4 oz/100 g) cottage cheese
Yoghurt/fromage frais	1 small pot (5 oz/150 g) yoghurt or fromage frais

◆ *Meat, fish and vegetarian alternatives* ◆

	Size of one portion
Meat	2 thin slices (2—3 oz/50—75 g) red meat 1 small chop (2—3 oz/50—75 g) 3 thin slices ham
Poultry	3 oz (75 g) chicken/turkey (weighed without bone) 1 small breast
Fish	1 medium fillet (5 oz/150 g) white fish 1 small fillet (3 oz/75 g) oily fish 1 small tin (4 oz/100 g) tuna 3—4 oz (75—100 g) prawns
Eggs	2
Pulses	Half a large (14 oz/400 g) tin baked beans/ red kidney beans/chick peas/other beans 3 heaped tbsp cooked beans/lentils/peas
Nuts	Small handful (2 oz/50 g) of nuts or seeds
Tofu/quorn	4 oz (100 g) tofu/quorn

◆ *Fats and oils* ◆

Size of one portion

Spreading fats 1 tsp butter/margarine
2 tsp low fat spread

Oils 1 tsp vegetable/olive oil

Dressings 1 tsp oil-based salad dressing (e.g. French dressing/mayonnaise)
1 tbsp salad cream

◆ *Fatty and sugary foods* ◆

Size of one portion

1 packet of crisps
1 slice of cake
3 biscuits
1 large scoop of ice cream
1 chocolate/confectionery bar

◆ Eating plan – 2000 calories ◆

	No of portions
Fruit	4
Vegetables	3
Cereals and starchy vegetables	9
Milk and dairy products	3
Meat, fish and vegetarian alternatives	2
Fats and oils	3
Fatty and sugary foods (optional)	1

Breakfast

Cereal

1 medium bowl (2 oz/50 g) wholegrain breakfast cereal (e.g. wheat flakes/bran flakes/Weetabix/shredded wheat/muesli/porridge oats) with ⅓ pint (200 ml) skimmed/semi skimmed milk; 1 piece of fruit or 1 glass (¼ pint/150 ml) fruit juice

OR

Toast

2 thick slices of wholemeal toast with 2 tsp butter/low fat spread; 1 glass (⅓ pint/200 ml) milk or 1 carton of yoghurt or 1 egg (boiled/scrambled)

Snack

1 piece of fruit or 1 glass (¼ pint/150 ml) fruit juice

OR

Small handful (1—2 oz/25—50 g) dried fruit (e.g. apricots, figs, raisins, dates)

Lunch

Sandwich

2 thick slices wholemeal bread or large wholemeal bap with 2 tsp low fat spread; 3 oz (75 g) tuna/chicken breast/cottage cheese or 1 oz (25 g) Cheddar or 1 tbsp peanut butter; 4 oz (100 g) salad with 1 tbsp dressing; 1 piece of fruit; 1 carton of yoghurt or fromage frais

OR

Baked potato

Medium jacket potato (6 oz/175 g) with 2 tsp low fat spread or butter; 3 oz (75 g) tuna/chicken breast/cottage cheese or 1 oz (25 g) Cheddar or half a tin (7 oz/200 g) baked beans; 4 oz (100 g) bowl of salad; 1 piece of fruit; 1 carton of yoghurt or fromage frais

OR

Hot or cold pasta

2 oz (50 g) pasta (uncooked weight) mixed with 3 oz (75 g) white fish/chicken breast/cooked beans/cottage cheese; 4 oz (100 g) mixed vegetables with 1 tbsp oil/vinegar dressing; 1 piece of fruit; 1 carton of yoghurt or fromage frais

OR

Hot or cold rice

2 oz (50 g) rice (uncooked weight) mixed with 3 oz (75 g) white fish/chicken breast/cooked beans/cottage cheese; 4 oz (100 g) peppers/tomatoes with 1 tbsp oil/vinegar dressing; 1 piece of fruit; 1 carton of yoghurt or fromage frais

Snack

6 rice cakes with 1 tbsp fruit spread

OR

2 slices of toast with 1 tbsp fruit spread

OR

1 oatbran or cornmeal muffin/wholemeal muffin/roll/small pitta/scone with 1 tbsp fruit spread

Supper

Pasta dish

3 oz (75 g) pasta or rice (uncooked weight); sauce made with tomatoes, peppers, mushrooms, 6 oz (175 g) cooked lentils or 3 oz (75 g) ham/poultry or 1oz (25 g) Cheddar cheese plus herbs cooked in 1 tsp olive oil; 3 tbsp vegetables (e.g. broccoli, courgettes); baked apple filled with 1 tbsp dried fruit plus ¼ pint (150ml) low fat custard or yoghurt

OR

Noodle stir fry

3 oz (75 g) noodles/rice; 3 oz (75 g) fish/poultry/seafood/tofu or 6 oz (175 g) cooked beans; 4 oz (100 g) vegetables stir fried in 1 tsp oil; 1 piece of fruit or fruit salad with 1 carton of fromage frais

OR

Jacket potato meal

1 large (9 oz/250 g) baked potato; 3 oz (75 g) chicken breast or 6 oz (175 g) cooked beans/lentil dahl; 4 oz (100 g) green vegetables; 4 oz (100 g) other vegetables; 4 oz (100 g) fresh fruit with 2 scoops of yoghurt ice

OR

Curry

3oz (75 g) fish/poultry/seafood/tofu/lean meat or 6 oz (175 g) cooked beans/lentils cooked with curry sauce and 8 oz (225 g) vegetables (e.g. onions, peppers, mushrooms, leeks, carrots, broccoli); 1 naan/chappati or 3 oz (75 g) rice; 3 tbsp yoghurt or raita; 4 oz (100 g) fresh fruit

OR

Low fat spaghetti bolognese

3 oz (75 g) spaghetti; sauce made with 3 oz (75 g) minced turkey or 6 oz (175 g) cooked lentils/red kidney beans plus onions, mushrooms, peppers; 4 oz (100 g) other vegetables; 4 oz (100 g) fresh or baked fruit

Optional snack

1 portion of fatty/sugary food

◆ Eating plan – 2500 calories ◆

	No of portions
Fruit	5
Vegetables	3
Cereals and starchy vegetables	12
Milk and dairy products	3
Meat, fish and vegetarian alternatives	2—3
Fats and oils	4
Fatty and sugary foods (optional)	1

Breakfast
Cereal
1 medium—large bowl (3 oz/75 g) wholegrain breakfast cereal (e.g. wheat flakes/bran flakes/Weetabix/shredded wheat/muesli/porridge oats) with ⅓ pint (200 ml) skimmed/semi skimmed milk; 1 piece of fruit or 1 glass (¼ pint/150 ml) fruit juice

OR

Toast
3 thick slices of wholemeal toast with 3 tsp butter/low fat spread; 1 glass (⅓ pint/200 ml) milk or 1 carton of yoghurt or 1 egg (boiled/scrambled)

Snack
2 pieces of fruit or 1 piece fruit and 1 glass (¼ pint/150 ml) fruit juice

OR

Small handful (2 oz/50 g) dried fruit (e.g. apricots, figs, raisins, dates)

Lunch
Sandwich
As for 2000 calories plan (*see* page 209).

OR

Baked potato
As for 2000 calories plan (*see* page 209).

OR

Hot or cold pasta
As for 2000 calories plan (*see* page 209).

OR

Hot or cold rice
As for 2000 calories plan (*see* page 209).

Snack
As for 2000 calories plan (*see* page 209).

Supper
Pasta dish
4 oz (100 g) pasta or rice (uncooked weight); sauce made with tomatoes, peppers, mushrooms, 8 oz (225 g) cooked lentils or 4 oz (100 g) ham/poultry or 2 oz (50 g) Cheddar cheese plus herbs cooked in 1 tsp olive oil; 3 tbsp vegetables e.g. broccoli, courgettes; baked apple filled with 1 tbsp dried fruit plus ¼ pint (150ml) low fat custard or yoghurt

OR

Noodle stir fry
4 oz (100 g) noodles/rice; 6 oz (175 g) fish/poultry/seafood/tofu or 8 oz (225 g) cooked beans; 4 oz (100 g) vegetables stir fried in 1 tsp oil; 1 piece of fruit or fruit salad with 1 carton of fromage frais

OR
Jacket potato meal
1 large (12 oz/350 g) baked potato; 4 oz (100 g) chicken breast or 8 oz (225 g) cooked beans/lentil dahl; 4 oz (100 g) green vegetables; 4 oz (100 g) other vegetables; 4oz (100g) fresh fruit with 2 scoops of yoghurt ice

OR
Curry
6 oz (175 g) fish/poultry/seafood/tofu or 4 oz (100 g) lean meat or 8 oz (225 g) cooked beans/lentils cooked with curry sauce and 8 oz (225 g) vegetables (e.g. onions, peppers, mushrooms, leeks, carrots, broccoli); 1 naan/chappati or 4 oz (100 g) rice; 3 tbsp yoghurt or raita; 4 oz (100 g) fresh fruit

OR
Low fat spaghetti bolognese
4 oz (100 g) spaghetti; sauce made with 4 oz (100 g) minced turkey or 8 oz (225 g) cooked lentils/red kidney beans plus onions, mushrooms, peppers; 4 oz (100 g) other vegetables; 4 oz (100 g) fresh or baked fruit

Optional snack
1 portion of fatty/sugary food

◆ Eating plan – 3000 calories ◆

	No of portions
Fruit	6
Vegetables	4
Cereals and starchy vegetables	15
Milk and dairy products	3—4
Meat, fish and vegetarian alternatives	3
Fats and oils	5
Fatty and sugary foods (optional)	1

Breakfast
Cereal
1 large bowl (4 oz/100 g) wholegrain breakfast cereal (e.g. wheat flakes/bran flakes/Weetabix/shredded wheat/muesli/porridge oats) with ⅔ pint (375 ml) skimmed/semi skimmed milk; 1 piece of fruit or 1 glass (¼ pint/150 ml) fruit juice

OR

Toast
4 thick slices of wholemeal toast with 4 tsp butter/low fat spread; 1 large glass (⅔ pint/375 ml) milk or 2 cartons of yoghurt or 2 eggs (boiled/scrambled)

Snack
2 pieces of fruit or 1 piece of fruit and 1 glass (¼ pint/150ml) fruit juice, plus 1 slice of bread/toast or 3 rice cakes

OR

Small handful (2 oz/50 g) dried fruit (e.g. apricots, figs, raisins, dates), plus 1 slice of bread/toast or 3 rice cakes

Lunch
Sandwich
4 thick slices wholemeal bread or 2 large wholemeal baps with 2 tsp low fat spread; 4 oz (100 g) tuna/chicken breast/cottage cheese or 2 oz (50 g) Cheddar cheese or 2 tbsp peanut butter; 4 oz (100 g) salad with 1 tbsp dressing; 1 piece of fruit; 1 carton of yoghurt or fromage frais

OR

Baked potato
Large jacket potato (9 oz/250 g) with 2 tsp low fat spread or butter; 4 oz (100 g) tuna/chicken breast/cottage cheese or 2 oz (50 g) Cheddar cheese or ¾ of a tin (11 oz/300 g) baked beans; 4 oz (100 g) bowl of salad; 1 piece of fruit; 1 carton of yoghurt or fromage frais

OR

Hot or cold pasta
3 oz (75 g) pasta (uncooked weight) mixed with 4 oz (100 g) white fish/chicken breast/cooked beans/cottage cheese; 4 oz (100 g) mixed vegetables with 1 tbsp oil/vinegar dressing; 1 piece of fruit; 1 carton of yoghurt or fromage frais

OR

Hot or cold rice
3 oz (75 g) rice (uncooked weight) mixed with 4 oz (100 g) white fish/chicken breast/cooked beans/cottage cheese; 4 oz (100 g) peppers/tomatoes with 1 tbsp oil/vinegar dressing; 1 piece of fruit; 1 carton of yoghurt or fromage frais

Snack
6 rice cakes with 1 tbsp fruit spread, plus 1 piece fruit

OR

2 slices of toast with 1 tbsp fruit spread, plus 1 piece fruit

OR

1 oatbran or cornmeal muffin/wholemeal muffin/roll/small pitta/scone with 1 tbsp fruit spread, plus 1 piece fruit

Supper
Pasta dish
As for 2500 calories plan (*see* page 211).

OR
Noodle stir fry
As for 2500 calories plan (*see* page 211).

OR
Jacket potato meal
As for 2500 calories plan (*see* page 212).

OR
Curry
As for 2500 calories plan (*see* page 212).

OR
Low fat spaghetti bolognese
As for 2500 calories plan (*see* page 212).

Optional snack
1 portion of fatty/sugary food

◆ Eating plan – 3500 calories ◆

	No of portions
Fruit	6
Vegetables	4
Cereals and starchy vegetables	18
Milk and dairy products	4
Meat, fish and vegetarian alternatives	3
Fats and oils	6
Fatty and sugary foods (optional)	1

Breakfast
Cereal
1 large bowl (4 oz/100 g) wholegrain breakfast cereal (e.g. wheat flakes/bran flakes/Weetabix/shredded wheat/muesli/porridge oats) with ⅔ pint (375 ml) skimmed/semi skimmed milk; 1 piece of fruit or 1 glass (¼ pint/150 ml) fruit juice plus 1 slice of toast with 1 tsp low fat spread and honey

OR

Toast
5 thick slices of wholemeal toast with 5 tsp butter/low fat spread; 1 large glass (⅔ pint/375 ml) milk or 2 cartons of yoghurt or 2 eggs (boiled/scrambled)

Snack
2 pieces of fruit or 1 piece of fruit and 1 glass (¼ pint/150ml) fruit juice plus 2 slices bread/toast or 6 rice cakes

OR

Small handful (2 oz/50 g) dried fruit (e.g. apricots, figs, raisins, dates) plus 2 slices of bread/toast or 6 rice cakes

Lunch
Sandwich
As for 3000 calories plan (*see* page 213).

OR

Baked potato
As for 3000 calories plan (*see* page 213).

OR

Hot or cold pasta
As for 3000 calories plan (*see* page 213).

OR

Hot or cold rice
As for 3000 calories plan (*see* page 213).

Snack
As for 3000 calories plan (*see* page 213).

Supper
Pasta dish
5 oz (150 g) pasta or rice (uncooked weight); sauce made with tomatoes, peppers, mushrooms, 8 oz (225 g) cooked lentils or 4 oz (100 g) ham/poultry or 2oz (50 g) Cheddar cheese plus herbs cooked in 1 tsp olive oil; 3 tbsp vegetables e.g. broccoli, courgettes; baked apple filled with 1 tbsp dried fruit plus ¼ pint (150 ml) low fat custard or yoghurt

OR

Noodle stir fry
5 oz (150 g) noodles/rice; 6 oz (175 g) fish/poultry/seafood/tofu or 8 oz (225 g) cooked beans; 4 oz (100 g) vegetables stir fried in 1 tsp oil; 1 piece of fruit or fruit salad with 1 carton of fromage frais

OR

Jacket potato meal
2 large (7 oz/200 g) baked potatoes; 4 oz (100 g) chicken breast or 8 oz (225 g) cooked beans/lentil dahl; 4 oz (100 g) green vegetables; 4 oz (100 g) other vegetables; 4oz (100g) fresh fruit with 2 scoops of yoghurt ice

OR
Curry
6 oz (175 g) fish/poultry/seafood/tofu or 4 oz (100 g) lean meat or 8 oz (225 g) cooked beans/lentils cooked with curry sauce and 8 oz (225 g) vegetables (e.g. onions, peppers, mushrooms, leeks, carrots, broccoli); 1—2 naan/chappati or 5 oz (150 g) rice; 3 tbsp yoghurt or raita; 4 oz (100 g) fresh fruit

OR
Low fat spaghetti bolognese
5 oz (150 g) spaghetti; sauce made with 4 oz (100 g) minced turkey or 8 oz (225 g) cooked lentils/red kidney beans plus onions, mushrooms, peppers; 4 oz (100 g) other vegetables; 4 oz (100 g) fresh or baked fruit

Optional snack
1 portion of fatty/sugary food

◆ Eating plan – 4000 calories ◆

	No of portions
Fruit	7
Vegetables	4
Cereals and starchy vegetables	21
Milk and dairy products	4
Meat, fish and vegetarian alternatives	3—4
Fats and oils	7
Fatty and sugary foods (optional)	1

Breakfast
Cereal
1 large bowl (4 oz/100 g) wholegrain breakfast cereal (e.g. wheat flakes/bran flakes/Weetabix/shredded wheat/Muesli/porridge oats) with ⅔ pint (375 ml) skimmed/semi skimmed milk; 1 piece of fruit or 1 glass (¼ pint/150 ml) fruit juice plus 2 slices of toast with 2 tsp low fat spread and honey

OR

Toast
6 thick slices of wholemeal toast with 6 tsp butter/low fat spread; 1 large glass (⅔ pint/375 ml) milk or 2 cartons of yoghurt or 2 eggs (boiled/scrambled)

Snack
As for 3500 calories plan (*see* page 215).

Lunch
Sandwich
6 thick slices wholemeal bread or 3 large wholemeal baps with 2 tsp low fat spread; 6 oz (175 g) tuna/chicken breast/cottage cheese or 3 oz (75 g) Cheddar cheese or 3 tbsp peanut butter; 4 oz (100 g) salad with 1 tbsp dressing; 2 pieces of fruit; 1 carton of yoghurt or fromage frais

OR

Baked potato
2 large jacket potatoes (6 oz/175 g) with 2 tsp low fat spread or butter; 6 oz (175 g) tuna/chicken breast/cottage cheese or 3 oz (75 g) Cheddar cheese or 1 tin (14 oz/400 g) baked beans; 4 oz (100 g) bowl of salad; 2 pieces of fruit; 1 carton of yoghurt or fromage frais

OR

Hot or cold pasta
6 oz (175 g) pasta (uncooked weight) mixed with 6 oz (175 g) white fish/chicken breast/cooked beans/cottage cheese; 4 oz (100 g) mixed vegetables with 1 tbsp oil/vinegar dressing; 2 pieces of fruit; 1 carton of yoghurt or fromage frais

OR

Hot or cold rice
6 oz (175 g) rice (uncooked weight) mixed with 6 oz (175 g) white fish/chicken breast/cooked beans/cottage cheese; 4 oz (100 g) peppers/tomatoes with 1 tbsp oil/vinegar dressing; 2 pieces of fruit; 1 carton of yoghurt or fromage frais

Snack
As for 3000 and 3500 calories plans (*see* page 213).

Supper
Pasta dish
As for 3500 calories plan (*see* page 215).

OR

Noodle stir fry
As for 3500 calories plan (*see* page 215).

OR

Jacket potato meal
As for 3500 calories plan (*see* page 215).
OR
Curry
As for 3500 calories plan (*see* page 216).
OR
Low fat spaghetti bolognese
As for 3500 calories plan (*see* page 216).

Optional snack
1 portion of fatty/sugary food

Index